There's No Good Book For This

But I Wrote One Anyway

The Irreverent Guide To Crushing Breast Cancer

Cara Lockwood

A note to readers

I hold no medical degrees, nor am I a licensed psychologist, and this book should not be a substitute for medical, legal, or financial advice.

This book is a part-memoir, and it's my present recollection of events as I remember them, and some events have been compressed and dialogue recreated. Also, sidenote: I'm a fifty-something, menopausal woman post cancer treatment, so my memory is shot. I did the best I could.

This is my lived experience, so it is unique to me. Your experience will be yours. There is certainly triggering material in these pages since everything about breast cancer is triggering because it's freakin' cancer. Read the chapter titles carefully, as they'll let you know about potentially upsetting content. Don't want to read about surgery? Skip Chapter Eleven. Hate thinking about chemo? Chapter Twelve is not for you.

Don't want to read about any details at all? Skip to the pep talks at the end of each chapter.

This book may not be your cup of tea, and that's fine. There is profanity in it, because... cancer. Everyone handles this battle differently, and what helps one person might not help another. What one person finds funny, another will absolutely not. We are all unique individuals, and nobody's battle is quite the same.

All, I can say is, for all of you in the fight of your lives, I see you. I've been where you are. This fight will wear you out. It will test the limits of your patience, your strength, and your sanity.

You'll dig deep and find reserves you never even knew were there.

I see you. I salute you. Keep battling every day. You're worth every ounce of effort.

"You are braver than you believe, stronger than you seem, smarter than you think, and twice as beautiful as you'd ever imagined."

—A.A. Milne, *Winnie-the-Pooh*

Table of Contents

Introduction
No One Asked for This

"Love and laughter are two of the most important universal cancer treatments on the planet. Overdose on them."

—Tanya Masse

This is the one book you never wanted to read.

So, your friend/mom/sister/cousin/neighbor gave you this book. Or you bought it as a little gift for yourself.

I'm sorry.

I'm sorry because this isn't a bottle of tequila, and that's probably what you really want right now.

I'm sorry because you have breast cancer, or someone you love has breast cancer, and everything sucks. This book is not going to cheer you up; nothing on *fucking earth* can cheer you up because it's *CANCER*.

No book is going to change that. It sucks, no matter what stage it's in. It doesn't matter that treatments are so much better than they used to be (they're not a walk in the park, let's be frank). It sucks because your life has officially been turned upside down.

I wish I could take your cancer away and give it to someone we both hate, but that's not how this works. I also wish cancer would just get cancer and fucking die, but that's not how this works either.

I'm just going to do my best to make you feel better. I'm going to try to make some jokes. Why? Because laughter is the best medicine.

Actually, scratch that. Laughter is NOT the best medicine. Medicine is the best medicine, and please do not go telling your oncologist that some weirdo who wrote a book told you that you are going to mirth your way straight to good health, that you don't need chemo because all you need is a good stand-up special on Netflix.

That is not how this works.

Also, this is not a book endorsed by medical professionals. You've no doubt received your Terrifying Phonebook of Breast Cancer Information, given to you by your doctor or team or well-meaning aunt, where every time you open it you see something absolutely awful, like a diagram of a mastectomy. Or a five-page list of all the terrible side effects of chemotherapy.

This is not that kind of book either.

The Terrifying Phonebook is great. We need it sometimes. But sometimes, we just need someone to crack a totally inappropriate joke. Something to make us laugh because all of this is absolutely horrifyingly scary, and if we don't laugh, we'll shit ourselves with terror.

And nobody wants an adult diaper full of that.

I want you to know: It's okay to be terrified. This shit is scary. Cancer kills people. It might not be the star of any true crime podcast, but that messy bitch is a straight-up serial killer. Cancer killed ten *million* people in the world in 2020. That accounts for 1 out of 6 deaths worldwide.[1]

So, it's okay to be scared. It's also okay to be furious. How did this even fucking happen?! Why me? Why the hell did I use all that overpriced organic deodorant if it didn't even prevent cancer?! It's okay to pout, to be petulant, and whine, WHY ME? It's okay to be sad. Because you've got a whole mountain ahead of you to climb. And you're wearing flip-flops.

---

[1] "Cancer Fact Sheet," World Health Organization, February 3, 2022.

I know what you're thinking. You're thinking I don't even walk on the beach well in flip-flops. How am I supposed to freakin' climb Mount Everest in them?

One step at a damn time.

One.

Lousy.

Wobbly.

Completely nongraceful.

I'm-sure-I'm-going-to-fall-on-my-ass.

Why am I wearing flipflops on a damn mountain? Did the airline lose my luggage. . . or am I just in the middle of the worst nightmare I've ever had. . . ? Also, I'm scared of heights!!

Step.

At.

A.

Time.

And that first step is this book.

Who is this bitch telling you about climbing mountains in foam soles? That's me. Hi. I'm Cara. I write under two names: Cara Lockwood (formerly married name) and Cara Tanamachi (the name my parents gave me). I'm a *USA Today* bestselling romance novelist, and I'm also a breast cancer survivor. I've been where you are. I've walked in plastic toe floss all the way from diagnosis to remission, so I know it can be done. I've got the blisters to prove it.

I was diagnosed with Stage 1, HER2+ invasive breast cancer in September 2023. Don't worry—my doctors said— you caught it early, thank God! Except that what they mean by "early" is that I would FUCKING live. It didn't mean the treatments were any less terrible. Over nearly sixteen months, I was the lucky recipient of: a double mastectomy, six weeks of physical therapy, one port insertion, twelve rounds of chemotherapy, twenty-six rounds of immunotherapy infusions, one reconstruction surgery, and a whole lot of swearing.

Now, I'm officially in remission.

That's great, you say. Good for you. Glad *you're* fine, but I'm not, and I'm petrified. Right now, you're in shock, or you're petrified, or you're in denial, or everyone you know is telling you that you've GOT THIS when you 100% DO NOT HAVE THIS and you're hiding in the shower bawling your eyes out. You're whiplashing back and forth between shock and terror, between avoidance and anger. You're bargaining. You're begging. You're trying to pray the cancer away. You're feeling every feeling on earth except acceptance.

I *get* it. This shit is terrifying. How do you even fight an enemy *that lives inside you*? I mean I battled insecurity my whole life and never made a dent in that asshole. If only body issues could kill cancer, my low self-esteem would've laid it out flat. If I could've mean-girled my way out of this diagnosis, I would've been all over it.

I know this post-diagnosis roller coaster is a ride you never signed up for, a path you never planned to take. This was not an intersection in your life that you wanted, not a label you planned for, not a trip you EVER wanted to go on. The attractions here are absolute shit. Restaurants? Terrible. Hotels? Good only if you liked being stabbed by needles *in your armpit* and wearing open-faced faded magenta smocks. Shopping? How does $2,000 for a single blood draw sound? One-star review—would NOT recommend.

Plan A was to never get breast cancer in the first place.

But, my friend, Plan A is a distant memory, and now you're here. Welcome to Plan B.

I'm going to be honest with you. I'm going to say completely inappropriate things. There truly IS no good book for this, but I wrote one anyway. Read it. Don't read it. Skip to the end. Let fate decide what you need to hear right now and open it straight in the middle. Use it as a paperweight. Light it on fire and scream at the flames. Whatever you need right now is what you need.

So, it's okay to be scared.

And it's okay to laugh.

It's especially okay to laugh. The best way to deal with fear is to laugh. It's hard to maintain shit-your-pants-inducing terror when you're laughing.

Not that any of this is funny.

Except some of it is.

I know you don't believe me.

But some of this can be funny. It can be funny because laughing at what scares us most is the very best way to make it *not* so damn scary anymore. Humor is LETHAL to fear. It cowers in front of a good joke. Gallow's humor? It's the only thing Death is scared of.

He's actually very thin-skinned and paranoid about people laughing in his face. So, let's point and laugh at him, shall we?

If we can make fun of something, we have power over it.

In middle school, a bully built like a linebacker targeted me and my friends. When she wanted to fight me, I hid in the nurse's office. BUT, I also relentlessly made fun of her until she wasn't so scary anymore.

I mean, I made fun of her behind her back. I'm no fool.

Laughing takes cancer's power away. We are going to bully the HELL out of cancer in this book. It deserves it.

A few notes about this book:

I refer to cancer as "she" and more often "that messy bitch," not to unfairly gender cancer, but because it started in my breast, and my breasts, in my mind, identify as she/her. Men get breast cancer, too, and they might have different pronouns for their cancer. And if my cancer started in my colon, that might be a he/him. Or they/them. I don't know.

I use profanity because, dammit, this is fucking cancer. They say using profanity makes you feel a little bit less pain, and I think you should have all the painkillers you can get right now.

I am not a medical professional or trained in any way and shouldn't be considered an expert on anything (ask my kids and they will 100% agree). I write romance novels for a living, and this is just my lived experience.

At the end of every chapter, I put in a pep talk because you'll need every fucking pep talk ever written. Skip to the end of every chapter if you just want a shot in the arm of positivity.

I cannot guarantee that everything will work for you, or me, or any of us. All we can do is what we can do. I'm going to share my story and tell you some things that worked for me. You are going to have to decide what works for you.

You're going to have to walk this road. I may or may not make you feel better, but I promise you this:

You are not alone.

Chapter One

Your New Normal
(Also, this Normal Sucks. WTF?!)

"You never know how strong you are until being strong is the only choice you have."

—Bob Marley

Welcome to the party, pal.

Hi. Welcome to the Newly Diagnosed Club. I'm not sure if it was today or last month when you first heard the news that your life had officially changed forever.

I will say to you what others who walked this path before me said:

Welcome to the worst club on earth. . . with the very best and strongest of members.

You are officially joining a club of badasses.

And I know you don't believe you belong here, but I promise you, you will rise to this occasion and dominate it. You will become a gold-armor-wearing gladiator who cuts their enemies down at the knees, who takes no prisoners, and who destroys anyone and anything that comes between you and the rest of your life. You will put some serious hurt on cancer, and you will get a hold of your fears, your worry, your anxiety, and your terror.

You know why?

The answer is simple.

Because you don't have a choice.

None of us in the Breast Cancer Warrior Club woke up one day and said, "Hey, what about this bravery thing? Let me give it a shot."

We didn't have a choice.

There must be some mistake.

"Cara? Hello. I've got the results of your biopsy," said the radiologist on the other end of the phone line as I stood in my kitchen between the as-yet-unloaded dishwasher and the sink full of dirty dishes I seriously meant to get to hours ago, cell phone pressed to my ear, half listening because I was already trying to think about what the hell I was going to make for dinner.

This was never an easy thing because we have a blended family of five children: three teens living with us and two twenty-somethings out in the wild. Among them: one vegetarian, one pescatarian, one carnivore, not to mention the one with tree nut allergies, one with peanut allergies, and one with both. And a whole wide array of preferences, none of which align.

Making dinner felt like entering the Thunderdome: seven people enter, and everyone leaves complaining. When my husband and I found a dish everyone would eat (jambalaya, for instance), then we'd make it so often they'd all hate it within three months.

If I ever won the lottery, I'd hire a full-time chef, or I'd simply let every child order what they want from DoorDash every single night.

"Yes?" Of course, I was eager to know the answer. Of course, I'd been slightly worried. But honestly, I wasn't really expecting bad news.

I wasn't supposed to get cancer. Nobody in my family had cancer, except my Japanese great-grandfather who died of throat cancer, but he smoked more than a pack a day. He smoked so much that my great-grandmother made artwork of a large crane made out of smaller origami cranes, folded from the shiny foil that lined his cigarette packs. She framed the artwork and it now takes up a large portion of my dad's dining room wall.

I mean, waste not, want not.

Most people in my family died of heart failure or strokes. High blood pressure and heart valve problems ran in my family. Strokes, sure. Everybody has a freakin' stroke. But cancer? Nobody got that. I was under the false impression that if I stayed fairly healthy and avoided cigarettes and other known carcinogens, I'd probably be fine. So, I dutifully scheduled my mammograms roughly every year, not because I was worried I'd get cancer, but because I fully expected them to be negative and benign.

It was just a box I checked because we all have that annoying friend/doctor/family member (I got mine this year, have you? HAVE YOU? [with pointed glare]). Okay, okay, I'll get my boobs squeezed! Happy now, perv?

I'd always needed two mammograms because I have dense breast tissue, so every year it was a scare. Every year they'd tell me my boobs were dense (it's a nice way of saying they weren't going to make the honor roll this year), and I needed to have a scary second mammogram, where they'd make me wait for instant results because it was all so dramatic.

Even the week before I got the results of my biopsy, I sat with friends on their patio, drinking a glass of wine on a warm fall evening and swatting away mosquitos, lamenting about how we all had dense breast tissue. How it was all such a *production*, and how it stressed us out, only to get a "You're all clear!" at the end.

I even talked about how my mother got dragged in and out of doctors' offices in the '80s and '90s for benign cysts that may or may not have been caused by hormones or caffeine or whatever, and she'd get scared to death every single time, only to be told, "Oops! Not cancer. No worries."

So, I was used to false alarms, and together, my friends and I were, too. We laughed about it and other indignities of being a middle-aged woman. We made jokes together because a man *almost definitely* invented the damn mammogram machine, and they would've made it better by now if *they* had to stick their testicles in it.

But then came the phone call about my biopsy results, with me absently opening the fridge door, glancing at the contents inside.

"The tumor is malignant," the radiologist said. "It's cancer."

As soon as he said the word, "cancer," my mind went blank.

Have you seen Season 3 of *Only Murders in the Building?* Steve Martin's character has to do this really complicated singing number for a new musical that Martin Short's character directs, and every time he tries, he gets stage fright. He just goes into a blank white room in his mind, while terrible things are happening in his reality.

The doctor said "cancer," and I marched straight into that white room, where the only sound I heard was a high-pitched whine, and I didn't hear anything else. I mean, I heard words. I held the phone to my ear; I nodded and made sounds like "Um-hmm" and "Oh." I pretended like I was there, but I wasn't. When I hung up, my husband, PJ, walked into the kitchen, asking who was on the phone. I said it was the doctor.

"What did he say?" PJ asked.

"Cancer."

"What? Seriously?" All the blood drained from PJ's face. He pulled me into his arms and hugged me.

"What stage is it?" he asked my hair.

"Uh. . . he said early?" What *did* he say again? I don't know.

"How early? Stage one?" PJ was getting more frantic, more upset, as he broke the hug.

"I don't know." I know the doctor said things. I couldn't remember a single thing.

"What do we do next?" he asked.

"I don't know." This was not like me not to know. I made it my business to know. I'm almost as Type A as you can get. I went to Penn—not Penn state, but the college Benjamin Franklin founded in Philadelphia in 1740.

I earned the achievement of being the only classmate of my Dallas suburban public high school class to get into the Ivy League because I worked hard, planned waaaaaaay far ahead, and did every single extracurricular activity my school had to offer.

I've published more than thirty-eight novels (and counting), dog paddling furiously to stay relevant in a publishing industry that LIVES to chew people up and spit them out. I always did the extra credit. I never left things to chance. The fact I didn't know what was happening goes to show exactly what kind of Mack truck had just run me over.

I'd been in the warm embrace of that blank white room. My mind had short-circuited, and my soul had left my body. I had no idea what the hell had just happened.

"He said something about precancerous and something about cancer." I seemed to remember that bit. Something about in situ, and whole bunch of jargon like I'd fallen onto the set of *Grey's Anatomy*, except there was only boring medical terminology and no hot doctors.

"Precancer?" P.J. sounded hopeful. "If it's just precancer, then it's not cancer, and maybe..."

"No, he said cancer. He definitely said cancer." I didn't go into the white room for a false alarm.

"Is it okay with you if I call him back and we ask questions?" P.J. was dying to call. He felt this must be some mistake, too. If we just talked to the manager, surely, we could get this all sorted out. I knew how he felt. I wanted this sorted out, too, because, again, I wasn't supposed to get cancer.

I nodded. Actually, I felt relieved. Yes, let's call back. Maybe I had heard wrong. I had been staring at the contents of my fridge wondering what the hell my kids would eat—can you have Mommy brain when your kids are fifteen and sixteen?

So, we called back. The doctor wasn't surprised we'd called back.

"This happens a lot," the doctor said.

I wasn't the only one who got waylaid in the white room then.

And it turned out, it wasn't precancer anything.

It was cancer, all right.

Malignant AF.

Cancer doesn't wait.

Cancer doesn't wait for your finances to be okay so you can pay your medical bills. It doesn't wait for your kids to be all set, not failing geometry, or for you and your in-laws not to be feuding. Cancer doesn't wait for you to get health insurance, or for you to—FINALLY—have that emergency fund saved. Cancer doesn't care if you're having a fight with your best friend, or if you've said yes to too many volunteer positions. It doesn't care if you've got anxiety or depression or if you're in a toxic relationship.

Cancer does not wait for you to have your shit together before it busts into your life.

Cancer does what it wants. When it wants. And what it wants is to *Kill You.*

Never forget that.

This isn't a courtesy call. Cancer isn't your friend.

THERE'S NO GOOD BOOK FOR THIS

Cancer is a messy bitch who lives for drama. If she lived outside your body, she'd make inappropriate, shady comments about your appearance to make herself feel better. She flirts with your spouse. She pines for her own season of *Real Housewives*. But if she got on the show, she'd get kicked off for "being too dramatic."

She's told you if your dad were single, she'd date him. For his money.

She calls you at two a.m. before your big final/work presentation/first day of work begging you to bail her out of jail. Again.

She came to your grandmother's funeral. High.

She borrowed your favorite necklace. And lost it.

She borrowed your favorite dress. And ruined it.

She borrowed your car. And totaled it.

Your parents don't like her. Your other friends don't like her. If she were any other person, she would've been kicked out of your friend group ages ago.

But when you try to end the friendship, she'll cry. And scream. And beg. And tell you she'll ruin your life if you ignore her.

Because no one just *ignores* her. You can't just *ignore* her. You can't just pretend she doesn't exist. The second you do, she's everywhere. All at once.

If you ignore her, she'll kill you.

So, you can't ignore her. You've got to poison her slowly, and then you've got to surgically cut her out of your life, and all the healthy borders around her that she even *touched* must be removed. You'll get her out of your life by confronting that bitch head-on. With everything you've got. You can't be *sort of* okay if she's in your life. You have to make it your mission to destroy every last trace of her.

Everyone has a horror story. But, the good news is, your horror story will be 100% unique to you.

So, here's what you'll find out: probably every single friend you know, almost every relative, will know someone who's had breast cancer.

One in eight women will get breast cancer in her lifetime. You will probably look around your friend group and say— shit, *I'm* the one. *I'm* the one who picked the short straw.

I know what you're thinking. One in *eight*, and my boob just jumped up and volunteered to be a tribute like this is the fucking *Hunger Games*?!

Yep, that's what just happened.

Despite feeling like your boob fell on a grenade to save the platoon, let me remind you that one in eight is a lot of fucking people. That means that almost everyone you know *knows* someone who's had breast cancer. Or is going through it.

Everyone will ask if you need to talk to a survivor or some-one who's going through it now; they can put you in touch. This is sweet. This can also be terrifying. Because the first time you talk to someone who is going through or survived breast cancer, you might hear the Whole Horrible Story.

And make no mistake: it is horrible.

But, remember, it might not be YOUR story.

The first thing you need to know is there are so many different kinds of breast cancer, and the treatments for each can be a little different. One person's experience isn't necessarily your experience. Yes, reach out, connect with people, talk, but only if you want to. Also know that whatever horror story they tell you, it might not be YOUR particular horror story.

So, you might be told chemo makes your fingernails fall out. Or that a mastectomy means you'll never feel your nipples again. Or worse, you won't have nipples at all, and you'll get to tattoo fake ones on. Yada, yada. These things are awful and true. For some. For many. But not all.

The good news is, my friend, that it's very possible your experience will probably be your own unique nightmare.

Congrats!

So, don't take on somebody else's horror show just yet. Yours will be its only very special kind of terrible.

You think there are common treatments like chemo, radiation, and surgery, but there are SO many kinds of each one, and so many unique combinations, that one person's story might not be your story at all. You might not even need chemo.

Or you might.

You might only get it once a month. Or once a week.

Just take a deep breath. No experience is 100% identical to another woman's experience. Your aunt's diagnosis is not your diagnosis. Every woman is different.

What is true is that it's too damn common.

One in eight women get it. That's more than 300,000 women a year.

Women are more likely to get breast cancer than any other cancer, and it mostly affects women fifty and older. We develop 83% of all new breast cancer cases, though like every fucking type of cancer more people are getting it earlier. If you're a Black woman, you're 4% less likely to develop cancer than a white woman, but 40% more likely to die from it.[2] Also, about 2,800 men are diagnosed with breast cancer every year; that comes out to 1 in 726 men who will develop breast cancer in their lifetimes.[3]

All those statistics 100% suck.

You'll soon discover that cancer is a messy bitch who has infiltrated the ranks when you weren't looking. Suddenly,

---

[2] Sandy McDowel, "Breast Cancer Death Rates Are Highest for Black Women—Again," American Cancer Society, October 3, 2022.
[3] "Key Statistics for Breast Cancer in Men," American Cancer Society, January 16, 2025.

people will come out of the woodwork—people you thought you knew well—who had cancer, or their sisters had it, or their mothers or aunts or coworkers.

They will overwhelm you with information. They will offer to talk. Do, don't, whatever you think will help. Honestly, some of them scared the shit out of me with horror stories of infections post-surgery or with nightmares around reconstruction, and I just wasn't ready for that. I didn't want to see anyone's scars. I didn't want to go to a support group. Hell, I had to give myself a pep talk just to go to the fucking doctor.

From the diagnosis on, there's going to be a whole lot of "Oh, shit, shit, shit. OH, SHIT. I am not ready for this." I am not ready for this treatment. I'm not ready for this biopsy. I'm not ready for this pain. I am JUST NOT FUCKING READY.

That's okay.

Take a deep breath.

You don't have to climb Mount Everest in flipflops in just *one* day. You'll have a little time to train for your ascent.

Also, remember that NOBODY is ready for this.

Who *plans* for cancer? Who gets *psyched up* for cancer?

NOBODY.

This shit is hard. And fucking terrifying.

This is a sucker punch. A curve ball nobody is prepared to hit.

All the warrior survivors in this damn club also sobbed in the shower and begged God or the universe for an easy way out. WE ALL DID. If you're not scared, if you're not looking for an escape route, then you're a sociopath with a weird genetic kink who does not properly fear pain or death.

So. The very first thing you need to do right now is be kind to yourself.

It's okay to freak out. It's okay to randomly start crying in your car. It's okay to bite your mother-in-law's head off when she not-so-politely implies this is all your fault because you didn't switch to aluminum-free deodorant. It's okay to rage against societal injustice and capitalism and uncaring insurance companies and deregulation and Red Dye 40 and everything else that is infuriating. It's okay to feel like there's no fucking way you're up for this battle.

You will be. You will.

Just not right now.

And it's okay not to feel ready.

This terrible time of a tailspin after diagnosis is horrible, but it won't last forever.

Nothing does.

So, keep reminding yourself of that.

This tailspin is temporary.

It's not forever.

You won't be in this free-fall from this diagnosis forever. You will get a handle on it. You'll figure out how you're going to fight it. Or hell, even if you're going to fight it. That, my dear, is your choice.

I can't make that decision for you.

All I can tell you is that this part, whatever part you're in, is temporary. Diagnosis, treatment, surgery—it's ALL temporary. It all will pass.

Whether it's dealing with the sucker punch of diagnosis, grappling with your treatment plan, recovering from surgery, battling through chemo, or nail-biting your way through radiation, the fear won't last. The treatments, if they stretch out for years or even for the rest of your life, won't be as terrifying as they are right now.

I promise you, the way you're feeling right now: off balance, off-kilter, like you can't find your footing? I promise you, that has an end date. That will end. We are going to get both those feet on the ground. You will get out of this tailspin.

Right now, you're skidding across the ice, feeling out of control, but you will steer into that damn skid and get your car back on the road. I promise.

You'll decide on a plan of action and then you'll execute that plan, and that part of this will be less terrifying, less stomach-dropping, than this part.

Hold on to that. Focus on that when things feel overwhelming. You don't have to hang on by your fingernails for all of eternity. You will get to solid ground again. It's coming.

So, take a deep breath. This category five tornado won't be on the ground forever.

You will get through the battery of tests. You will get a plan of treatment. You will decide what you're going to do about this messy bitch who's come into your life uninvited.

Cancer will go back to hell where it came from, and you'll send it there, screaming.

The Windowless Office with the Round Table

Let's talk about this damn room. Maybe this is not where you heard the bad news, but it's where I heard... Every. Single. Bad. Thing.

It's a small room at your oncologist/breast cancer surgeon/mammogram center's office with one round table with two to four chairs. It'd be the perfect size for three friends to catch up over coffee. But this doesn't have anything to do with lattes and gossip.

There are brochures on the table, or they're stacked neatly on the small desk in the corner (it's always in the corner), the desk with the computer on it. The doctor/nurse's/radiologist's desk. There's almost never a window. It's almost always a windowless office. Because if there were a window people would try to escape. It's probably been tried before.

There's never a sink, an exam table, or even a cabinet. Sometimes, there's a little bookshelf filled with books and brochures that you hoped never to have to read in your life. They're all about cancer.

There's almost never any pictures on the walls because someone couldn't decide whether wall art would add insult to injury. It probably would.

Desk. Computer. Round table. Chairs.

Is the table round because they don't want sharp edges in here? I don't know.

This is the room of Bad News. Test results here are malignant. Or there's a biopsy needed. It's the *This is further along than we thought* room. It's the *Ultrasound showed something suspicious* room. It's the *We don't think we can do a lumpectomy, it'll have to be a mastectomy* room.

It's the *It's not the news we were hoping for* room.

Nobody ever tells you good news in that room. You never learn you've won the lottery, your kids got a free scholarship to the college of their choice, or you just qualified for a zero-interest car loan. When you're in the room, you know it's bad.

I hate that fucking room.

I hate those fucking chairs.

I hate that fucking table with the helpful brochures on it.

I hate sitting at the table, in the windowless room, waiting for the bad news. And it feels like it's just always bad.

But, I need the information.

I need it because there's no way I can fight this enemy blind.

Don't Kill the Messenger

Here's the thing I want you to remember. Inside, you want to burn that room to the ground. You want to yell at the doctor/nurse navigator/radiologist in there. You want to blame them.

Don't.

I'm going to remind you now, and keep reminding you, that cancer is the asshole.

Cancer is the enemy. Don't let cancer divert or distract you. It is what you're fighting. Not your oncologist, the radiology tech who missed your vein, or the surgeon who's forty minutes late to an appointment.

Cancer is the enemy. Cancer is trying to kill you.

All you need to do is gather the people you think will best kick its ass. Don't take it out on The Helpers. If they're bad Helpers, find new ones.

And keep your eye on the enemy: it's cancer.

It's My Cancer Party and I Can Cry if I Want To

You're going to be knocked down. Cancer knocks everyone down. Nobody gets a cancer diagnosis and pops right back up and says, "Sweet. No worries. I got this."

If you are saying that, you're in denial, and there's an emotional freight train with your name on it that will flatten you at some point. Then you can come back to this section.

You will cry. You will rage. You will bargain. You will try to snuggle into the blanket of denial.

That's all just normal.

After I got my diagnosis, I spent some time at my Pity Party of One. Part of the first week was just shock. *I* can't have cancer. Cancer happens to Other People. It doesn't happen to me. I eat right! I gave up aluminum deodorant at age twenty-five. While I might smell like rotten patolli, that was the price I paid for being breast cancer free! I grit my teeth through nursing my kids because—hey, people who nurse lower their risks of developing cancer! I let the grays come in and didn't dye my hair!

I *put in the work* not to get cancer.

WTF?!

But cancer doesn't care.

So, let me tell you: have your pity party. It's okay. It's normal. Wallow in it, for a week. Maybe two. Every person I told during this time told me I'm a fighter and I got this, but I was a terrified wreck, and I absolutely DID NOT HAVE IT.

I wanted to hide under the covers and pretend none of it was happening. I was not up to this fight. I was scared. I was overwhelmed with the information. I feared making a decision or not making a decision.

I had just turned fifty and felt like facing down mortality was not fair. I thought I'd have more time. Why was this coming now? Why me? I didn't deserve this. I tried to be a good person. I thought I was lucky.

Had all my luck run out? Why me? Why was God/the universe punishing me? Is it because I'm a lapsed Methodist/ Protestant/Pretty Much Agnostic/Sometimes Atheist?

But I came to realize, why not me?

It didn't have anything to do with fault. Or whether or not I deserved it. Millions of women have breast cancer, and none of them deserves it.

None of them asked for it.

This isn't about punishment. Bad things happen to good people all the time. Good things happen to bad people – all the time.

Next, you might want to look for someone to blame. Pesticides. Hair dye. Baby powder. Genetically modified food. You can get angry at them all. But, don't let them distract you from the real fight. You've got PLENTY of time to be angry AFTER you've kicked cancer's ass.

If you rail against God, the universe, or capitalism too long, you'll forget who the real enemy is. It's cancer.

It's trying to fucking KILL you.

But you're not going to let it.

You can take up a sword against corporate greed or chemicals in our food/environment some other time.

Right now, you need to fight the army that's trying to put you in the ground. Think of it this way: the enemy is storming the gates, so you don't have the luxury of figuring out why. You have to fight the enemy who is trying to murder you right now.

And that's cancer.

Pep talk #1:

Hi. I see you. This sucks. You're thinking how can I possibly do anything? How can I even manage any of this? First thing's first— everything you're feeling is okay.

Feel all the feelings. Let them come and go. Nobody is prepared for this. Nobody handles this well, and even if they did, there are no medals for being calm.

Cancer is trying to kill you. She's a bitch. Are you going to hand cancer your life? Are you voluntarily putting your head in the guillotine? Fuck no, my friend.

Cancer is a messy bitch who lives for drama, but we will not let her win.

Right? Right!

Let's go kick cancer's ass.

Chapter Two

Face Your Fear—It's Not Going Away and Ignoring It Just Makes It Awkward

"It's about focusing on the fight and not the fright."

—Robin Roberts

You might think cancer is the most dangerous thing in your life right now, but actually, it's fear.

Let me tell you a little story about fear.

I grew up in the suburbs of Dallas to my Japanese American orthopedic surgeon dad and my Irish-Scottish American elementary school teacher mom. We did well for ourselves, and we were fortunate enough to have a kidney-shaped pool in our backyard. I lived in this pool even when it became hot bathwater in the Texas summers. Dad loved to complain about how much money we spent on said pool ("Want to know what it feels like to have a pool?" he'd joke. "Then go dig a hole in your yard and throw money in it.").

One unusually warm spring afternoon, Mom planned to have company that evening and busied herself cleaning the house. She sent me (then ten) and my little brother (then three) outside because she was tired of us undoing all the good cleaning she'd been doing with our sticky, smudgy fingers. We had on our good church clothes, and she told me in very strict terms not to let my brother—or I—get dirty. This meant that I could *not* climb up into my dusty tree house as I wanted, and I'd have to just hover and make sure my brother didn't decide today was the day to roll around in the dirt, which he did surprisingly often.

Matt made a beeline for his little, yellow mini motorized four-wheeler. It was a plug-in toy he'd gotten from Santa that same year and he LIVED on it. The thing went maybe just slightly slower than a ten-speed bike and he loved it. So he went straight to it, hopped on, and began buzzing around the pool. This was back in the '80s when nobody thought to put fences or gates up around pools, or any kind of guard rails, and we gave motorized vehicles to toddlers. We weeded out the weak by not wearing seatbelts or helmets and by jumping on trampolines without safety nets.

I yawned, bored, as I watched him, itching to go climb up in my treehouse, but knowing Mom would kill me if I did. I'd 100% get dirty, and besides, I was supposed to have eyes on Matt the whole time and his knees loved mud more than mine did.

I watched Matt take the corner around the deep end, past the diving board, but he turned the handlebars a little too sharply, his left wheel getting a little too close to the edge of the pool. Before I could even call out, the mini-four-wheeler and my brother fell straight into the crystal blue deep end.

I ran to the edge just in time to see the four-wheeler sink to the bottom. My brother popped up, brown eyes huge with fear, his mouth and nose bobbing above and beneath the water as he desperately tried to remember how to dog paddle. He'd only had maybe a summer of swim lessons and, as far as I knew, never swam without a kickboard. I'd already had years of swim lessons. I could lap the pool. I scooped up every weighted ring thrown to the bottom of the deep end. Fear slammed my chest. I had two directives: keep my brother out of trouble AND not get dirty. I was failing them both.

I kneeled at the edge of the pool and reached out a hand. "Matt! Grab my hand!"

He tried, the little guy. But he was too far out, and his arms were too short. Fear invaded every corner of my ten-year-old brain. Matt was drowning. Mom was going to kill me. How do I save him? Do I run back into the house and get Mom? Do I jump in and ruin my fancy clothes? But Mom said not to get dirty! What... What do I do? For a second, I just felt white-hot panic.

Panic. It can choke you. Especially when it seems like there's no good decision to be made. Panic took hold of me, pure fear, and it screamed at me to FLEE to run back into the house and get help. This problem was too big for me. I needed adult help. I needed Mom.

But then—for reasons I still don't understand now (maybe it was the universe, a higher power, whatever you believe in)—I hesitated. I took a breath. I just took a breath. And then my logical brain kicked on, and I looked into Matt's terrified eyes, as his nose and mouth sank beneath the water, his wet clothes and shoes pulling him down.

I stuffed down my fear, screaming at me to run to the house, because what I needed to do was jump in. To hell with getting dirty and ruining my outfit. Because when fear subsided and my logical brain kicked in, I realized there wasn't time to get Mom. The water was nearly to Matt's eyebrows. So, I jumped in. I grabbed Matt and tugged him to the side of the pool. I heaved him out. He got to his feet, soaking wet, coughing out water and scream-crying. He ran up the patio stairs to the back door, bawling, and I followed, dripping wet. I slid open the glass door and called for Mom, and she came, eyes bulging.

"What on earth? Cara, I *told* you..." she sputtered, furious.

"Matt fell in the pool!" I pointed back to the blue water. That's when Mom saw Matt's four-wheeler upside down at the bottom. And then everything became crystal clear, and she wasn't angry anymore. She was scared and relieved, as she clutched Matt to her chest in a very wet, chlorine-smelling hug.

Fear is an important emotion. It tells us when there's danger, and it tells us we need to act quickly to do something about it, but it can also cloud your thoughts and make it hard to come to a decision.

At the pool, I was lucky that I found a way to kick my logical brain on before my brother dipped below the surface of the water, and I was also lucky at age ten to have made the right decision. I hate to think what would've happened if I'd gone to get Mom, in that extra couple of minutes it would've taken to get help.

Cancer, however, is scarier than any damn pool.

Fear clouds your judgment.

Cancer is horrifying.

You have every reason to be afraid. We've gone over this. You thought you had plenty of time to worry about your own mortality but surprise! Time's up. It's NOW, bitch. You thought you had decades to get comfortable with dying? Try months or even weeks!

You're thirty or forty or fifty or sixty or seventy. It doesn't matter your age because none of us think about death until Death shows up on our doorstep and *makes* us think about him. Ding-ding, time's up! While everyone else is living their lives, blithely not worried about death, you've got the grim reaper crowding up your life like a tailgater on the freeway.

Fear is a natural response to your doctor telling you that you could literally DIE. That your body is trying to kill you in the worst of ways. Fear will strangle your logical brain. That's what it's designed to do.

Fear paralyzes you. Fear lies to you. Fear bullies you. Fear grabs hold of your heart with icy-cold fingers and won't let go. Fear convinces you that you already have one foot in the grave so why try? Fear turns you into a raging asshole, who blames everyone in your family and everyone you meet because they don't have cancer and you do.

Ignore the fear and it gets bigger. Deny it exists and it rears its ugly head in the middle of a performance review, a parent-teacher conference, or in line at the grocery store. It will keep you staring at the ceiling at three in the morning or stuffing your face with everything from the fridge, morning, noon, and night. Ignore fear and it will wreak havoc in your life, making everything worse.

You can't ignore the fear forever, and the fastest, best way to get a handle on it is to call it out. Fear is the original bully, and the only way to deflate its power is by facing it. Facing it might seem like the scariest thing there is, but trust me, it isn't. Fear isn't real. It's just noise. Fear is your body trying to keep you alive. When we were all Neanderthals fighting saber-toothed tigers, fear was great. Fear got the adrenaline pumping and we could run or fight that tiger with the terrible overbite. We survived, and so we passed down fear because it's a great survival tool.

But fear doesn't help you fight cancer.

You don't need a burst of adrenaline to outrun a saber-tooth.

You need calm, collective thinking. You need clarity, decisiveness, and confidence. You need to control your anxiety, not have your anxiety control you. You need to be able to hear someone tell you, "Everything happens for a reason," and not strangle the life out of them. You need to not freak out inside the MRI machine when it sounds like Jason is hacking at the thing with an axe.

So.

Instead of succumbing to fear, just take a breath. Take a big breath. Exhale. Let your logical brain come back online.

Fear is irrational.

I've talked to cancer survivors who were more afraid of losing their hair than of dying.

This is just fact.

You might be one of these people.

You might fear losing your hair or your breasts more than you fear losing your life. You fear a change in your appearance will devastate you forever. It's not an uncommon concern. Some women say they cried more when they lost their hair than when they got the cancer diagnosis. I'm sure this has nothing to do with the fact that we're told since we're little girls that our appearance is really all that matters.[4]

Straight, cis men are not told this. Men do not, as a rule, consider opting out of life-saving chemo because they might lose their hair. Women do because we're told our appearance is the most valuable thing about us. We're told that our very social status depends on the way we look.

If you really think about it, I'm sure you know that you are more than just what you look like. I am going to spell it out just in case: your appearance is the LEAST important thing about you. Your mind, heart, and spirit—the way you show up for people in your life, the way you love and care for those in your circle, the kick-ass way you tackle your workload? These attributes are far more important than whether you have eyebrows—or not.

Before you opt out of treatment and to go to your grave with all your luscious locks, I implore you to dig deeper into yourself.

What ARE you afraid of?

---

[4] Andrew A. Nelson and Christia Spears Brown, "Too Pretty for Homework: Sexualized Gender Stereotypes Predict Academic Attitudes for Gender-Typical Early Adolescent Girls," *Sage Journal*, May 23, 2018.

Rejection? From whom? Your spouse? Your friends or family? What's driving your fear of losing your hair or changing your appearance?

In cave dweller times, rejection from the group meant death, and many of us fear social rejection like we fear a stray bullet. Because, historically, rejection from the cave meant almost certain doom, and not just any kind of death—a painful and lonely death. Even today, rejection can hurt as much as a physical injury.[5]

We're hard-wired to avoid rejection as much as we'd avoid a broken arm.

But—it's time for our logical brains to kick back on. In modern times, rejection from society doesn't mean death.

And, spoiler alert, you won't be rejected from society because you LOSE YOUR HAIR WHILE FIGHTING FUCKING CANCER.

What kind of ginormous asshole mocks your bald head when you have breast cancer? THAT asshole will be soundly rejected by the group. Nobody expects you to win a beauty pageant when you're fighting cancer.

People will admire your strength and resilience—two attributes that aren't just skin deep.

So, I implore you, study your fear. Dig deep into it. What are you afraid of?

Being embarrassed?

You HAVE FUCKING CANCER. CANCER should be embarrassed. NOT you.

Feeling ugly?

Did Joan of Arc worry about what she looked like when she was slicing down her enemy on the battlefield? I think not.

Worried about your spouse finding you ugly?

---

[5] Kirsten Weir, "The pain of social rejection as far as the brain is concerned, a broken heart may not be so different from a broken arm," American Psychological Association, April 2012.

Would YOU reject your spouse if they lost their arm?

I cannot tell you this enough: fear lies to you. It tells you you'll die of embarrassment (you won't). It tells you no one will love you (the good ones always love you, no matter what). It tells you people will ridicule you (Who? The ginormous asshole? Yeah, who gives a shit what he thinks?). It tells you that you should be embarrassed you got cancer (Why? Because you're the unlucky one of eight women in America who will? You didn't CHOOSE cancer).

Fear lies. Fear is the ultimate unreliable narrator. Do not believe what fear tells you.

Fear doesn't care about the stats.

I've got good news for you. From 1989 to 2020, the death rates from breast cancer went down forty-three percent (the death rates didn't go down as fast for most women of color because of systemic discrimination and disparities of care—but they still did go down). So fewer women are dying of breast cancer than ever before. Your survival rate just went UP.

But fear doesn't care about that. Fear doesn't care that you're more likely to survive now than if you'd gotten the same diagnosis in the '80s.[6] Fear doesn't care.

Inhale. Exhale. Breathe out the fear.

I know this feels impossible in the moment. But remember this. Here's the thing about fear: fear ISN'T real. Fear is imaging the worst-case scenarios have already occurred, but they haven't. Fear can't hurt you. Fear can only manipulate

[6] Angela N. Giaquinto MSPH, Hyuna Sung Ph.D, Kimberly D. Miller MPH, Joan L. Kramer MD, Lisa A. Newman MD, MPH, Adair Minihan MPHA, Ahmedin Jemal DVM, Ph.D, Rebecca L. Siegel MPH, "Breast Cancer Statistics, 2022," CA: *A Cancer Journal for Clinicians*, October 3, 2022.

you and make you say insensitive things to the scheduling nurse. Fear might make you snap at the kids and tell them to do their own damn laundry. Fear makes you want to keep it all secret and soldier on alone, even though, friend, nobody gets a medal for that (see Chapter Five: Martyrs Die Alone. Don't Be A Martyr.).

But fear feels overwhelming. It short-circuits the nervous system and hijacks the brain because *that's what it was designed to do.*

The smartest parts of our brain shut down so we can focus on rapid responses.[7]

If you were facing a saber-tooth, you certainly wouldn't want fear to take a backseat to being distracted by whether or not you left the fire burning back at the cave. Of course, you'd want the fear to slap you across the face and tell you to *Run, dummy. There's a saber-toothed tiger that's planning to eat you for dinner!*

So how do we short-circuit fear? How do we wrestle back control of our brain from the very thing designed to keep us alive for millennia?

It starts with a change of focus, and that means understanding a few basic truths:

1. Cancer Doesn't Get to Decide.

You might feel like cancer has busted into your life and taken the wheel, that everything is about that messy bitch who lives for drama and you are no longer in control. I know I did.

But this is a lie.

You might feel that cancer has ALL the power, and you have none.

This is also a lie.

---

[7] Maia Szalavitz, "How Terror Hijacks the Brain," *Time Magazine*, April 16, 2023.

You might feel like cancer is the predator, and you're the victim, that you have no hope of any normal life again and you're now at the whim of the callous, spiteful master, cancer.

This is a lie.

Cancer is not your master.

Cancer doesn't have the power.

Cancer doesn't get to decide.

Cancer is a toddler throwing a tantrum in Target, but cancer doesn't run your life.

You are the grown-up running your own life, and you won't be sidetracked by cancer's immature antics.

It doesn't get to decide your treatment.

It doesn't get to decide your attitude.

It doesn't get to decide how you live your fucking life.

YOU get to decide.

Doctors don't get to decide either. Neither does your spouse. Or your kids. Or your friends.

You get to decide.

You will talk to the doctors. You will go down a deep rabbit hole online of alternative medicine. You will weigh your options. You'll probably lie awake at night worrying about them.

But YOU will decide.

You might get some treatment. You might decline some treatment.

It's YOUR choice.

Not cancer's. Not anyone else's.

Fuck cancer. That messy bitch has had enough say. She doesn't get to decide anything.

You'll decide what treatment you'll get. You'll decide where you'll get your treatment. You'll decide how you feel about it.

Cancer doesn't get to decide.

And, by the way, neither does anyone else.

Your body, your choice, my friend.

YOU are driving this bus. You are the captain of this ship. No one else.

This is very important to wrap your head around. Especially when you feel powerless. Especially when you feel like a victim. Especially when you want to throw up your hands, give up, and just let cancer steer your life.

You still have the power. Cancer doesn't have the power.

You are going to cut it out, radiate it out, poison it, or you're going to organically granola the thing to death.

You have the power.

Cancer doesn't get to decide.

Keep reminding yourself of this, over and over again. Because breast cancer is a messy bitch who lives for drama and will start bossing you around. Don't let her. Ultimately, the treatment course you take (surgery, no surgery, lumpectomy, mastectomy, chemo, no chemo, radiation, no radiation) is YOUR decision.

2. You can be a victim. Or you can be a survivor.

When scary things happen to us, we can typically take two approaches to it: we can feel that there's something we can do about it, or we feel that everything is out of our control.

Psychologists refer to this as Locus of Control. We, as humans, typically fall into two camps: those who have more of an internal locus of control and external locus of control folks. Internal locus of control are people who believe they write their own destiny. External locus of control people feel they are complete victims to chance and can do nothing to change their fate.[8] Many of us fall on the spectrum—feeling we can change some things but can't change others.

As you might guess, those who feel they have some control over their destinies feel more confident and are more self-

---

[8] "Locus of Control," *Psychology Today.*

sufficient than those who feel they are simply being batted around by the winds of fate. The good news is that we can all learn to take more control over our attitudes and lives and, over time, start to feel less like victims.

Cancer, in particular, would LOVE it if you wallowed in victimhood. It would love it if you sat around and did nothing to fight it, just wanting to be consoled twenty-four-seven. Get the fainting salts! Meanwhile, cancer will grow and thrive.

Look, later on in your life you can be a damsel in distress, but right now we need Wonder Woman to come stomp cancer's ass, which won't happen if fear is telling you that you're helpless, you're a victim, and nothing can be done about it.

Despite the lies fear and cancer are telling you, you do have a choice about how to handle this.

You can be a victim. Or you can be a survivor.

You can let cancer take down your mind long, long before it takes down your body. Or you can decide that you won't let it take up free real estate there.

So—be a survivor.

Survivor sounds cheesy. Do we need to cue "Eye of the Tiger" right now?

Maybe.

I know what you're thinking. Does this mean you're going to be one of those annoying cancer survivors who talk endlessly about organic kale shakes and quinoa, that bullies friends into doing a sixty-mile Susan G. Komen walk wearing pink feather boas and sparkly tutus?

Possibly.

You might be that annoying. You might plaster your car with bumper stickers. Or pester your coworkers to donate to cancer research. Or bully all your friends to get mammograms, regardless of their age or health insurance status.

Yes, you might become THAT person. The one who shows strangers in elevators their cancer survival tattoo. Across their whole chest. Or their forehead. Who cares where?

You might be the one who puts pink ribbons in her yard, hands them out at Halloween, or bugs the PTA endlessly to run a fundraiser in October.

But that will be awesome, and do you know why?

Because YOU'LL BE ALIVE.

You'll be alive to be absolutely intolerable to all your friends. You'll wear more pink than Barbie every fucking day in October and talk NONSTOP about your double mastectomy. You'll dress up as a giant pink ribbon for Halloween. You'll warn people in airports to get all their screenings because you're a walking cautionary tale. People will run from you.

But it will be awesome.

Because you'll be alive. And being alive means you've earned the right to be as damn annoying as you want.

3. Shitty Attitudes Make for Shitty Results, so Your Outlook Matters

When it comes to surgery, if you think you're going to do poorly, you will. If you think you are strong and will do well,—you WILL.[9]

I hate to break it to you, Glass Half Empty, but if you go in with a woe-is-me attitude, cancer is going to clean your clock.

"What you think, you become," the Buddha said. I'm not going to get into meditating or vibing with the universe or the power of attraction or any of that new-age stuff, but I'll just say

---

[9] Jennifer Waljee, Evan P McGlinn, Erika Davis Sears, Kevin C Chung "Patient expectations and patient-reported outcomes in surgery: A systematic review," *Surgery*, May 2014.

this: cancer might be trying a hostile takeover of your body, but do not let it take your soul.

You can worry. You can be afraid. That's not what I mean by a shitty attitude. You can't help but be worried and be freakin' terrified. A bad attitude kind of looks like this: *These treatments will never work. Nothing will work.*

It's deciding you've lost before you even step on the battlefield. Don't tell yourself you have no chance, that you're weak, that you can't do this, before you even give yourself the chance to try.

Your attitude – whether you believe you can or you can't – is an essential part of your arsenal.

4. Fear is turbulence, not the plane crash.

One of my favorite songs about fear is P!nk's "Turbulence." In it, it's clear she says fear tells you the plane has already crashed. Fear tells you you're already dead. It's petrifying.

But fear is just turbulence. That's all it is.

The plane hasn't crashed. You're going through some bumpy air. That's all. Don't crash the plane in your head before you even get a chance to try landing it.

There's also a fantastic quote from *Dune*. Yes, bitch, I am quoting *sci-fi* at you right now. That's how dire the situation is. I'm pulling out freakin' *Frank Herbert* quotes. Next it will be J.R.R. Tolkien. Do not mess with my inner nerd.

Okay, so the quote is this:

> I must not fear. Fear is the mind-killer. Fear is the little-death that brings total obliteration. I will face my fear. I will permit it to pass over me and through me. And when it has gone past I will turn the inner eye to see its path. Where the fear has gone there will be nothing. Only I will remain.

Fear is the mind-killer. Because fear short-circuits your brain. When you feel fear, *feel it, acknowledge it*. See it. Know it. It's fear. It's loud. It's making a lot of ruckus. But it's a storm that blows over you. Once the fear rants and raves and washes over you, then you'll see it's just noise. You'll still be there. You're still alive. The plane hasn't crashed.

I'm fucking terrified and none of this is helping.

Yeah. I get it. The first few weeks after diagnosis, I felt like I was having a heart attack. All the time. Every day. Fear shadowed me everywhere I went.

I was terrified. Part of this terror is all about the uncertainty, the not knowing about how bad the cancer is, or what kind of treatment plan you'll get. The fear is the worst right now, but fear will hang around for a long while. The fear doesn't go away. Bravery is doing something EVEN THOUGH you're scared shitless. You know you're brave because you will be fucking terrified.

Period.

So, it's just important to acknowledge it. See it. Know it's there (and, believe me, you'll know it when you wake up in the middle of the night and your heart is racing).

Everyone in this breast cancer club knows fear.

Someone said when you're doing bravery right it feels like fear.

You know what? It does.

Being brave just means that you keep on going, even when you're scared. Especially when you're scared.

Fear is a barking dog.

I have an amazing dog—a ninety-five-pound goldendoodle with a heart of gold, Teddy Bear.

Ted barks with the same ferocity at an UPS truck that he does at a coyote loose in the yard. He's got one volume: loud.

So does fear.

Fear is trying to keep you alive. We fear many things. We fear that saber-toothed tiger. We also fear being shunned and rejected. We fear pain. We fear all kinds of things.

But the bark is the same. It's loud. It's insistent.

Acknowledge the bark.

Acknowledge the fear.

Let it wash over you.

Do what I do when Teddy barks. I thank him for letting me know about the UPS truck, about the guy walking his chihuahua, about the bird that landed on the shrub in front of the window. *Thank you. I hear you.* And then I move on.

Because you're going to be a survivor, not a victim. You're not going to let cancer decide. You're going to take your power back.

Pep talk #2:

Hey there, friend. This time is scary. Does it feel like fear has a chokehold on you all the time?

Remember, fear is the turbulence, not the plane crash.

It's the dog barking at the UPS delivery person outside, not an actual burglar in your house.

Fear is noise. And it makes a lot of noise.

Listen to it. Acknowledge it. Pat it on the head, and let it wash over you, and drain away.

You'll need to be clear-headed for the fight ahead, and that means not being distracted by fear.

In your darkest moments, I want you to remember Cancer Doesn't Get To Decide. You're driving this bus (even if you never wanted to drive), and YOU get to decide what treatment you get. Cancer doesn't get to decide, and fear doesn't get to decide, either.

You—your rational self—gets to decide to be a survivor or a victim, and I already know you're a survivor.

You've got what it takes to survive deep in you. It's what kept your ancestors alive for thousands of years.

You're not here by accident.
And staying here with us won't be an accident either.
The fight is in you.
It's always been in you.

Chapter Three

Getting a Plan of Care—Welcome to Your New Role as a Human Pincushion

"Cancer didn't bring me to my knees, it brought me to my feet."

—Michael Douglas

If you're at the newly diagnosed stage, you (and your doctors) probably don't know what the hell is really happening in your body. You know it's cancer, but how far along? What can I do to treat it? At this stage, they're still finding all that out.

Your journey as a Human Pincushion has just begun.

This is the stage where doctors run a whole bunch of tests, usually involving needles of varying kinds. You get drips and drabs of information, and no confirmation whatsoever about your course of treatment. These are the worst if/then logic SAT problems in the world:

If this biopsy is clear, then surgery.
If this biopsy isn't, then chemo.
If this MRI is clear, then surgery.
If it's not, then chemo.
Maybe chemo, surgery, radiation.
Lions, tigers, and bears—oh, my!

And on and on and on. At this stage of diagnosis, you'll get so fucking tired of that small room with the round table and chairs that you will beg to have news delivered to you in the elevator.

I'm not going to say this is the *worst* part of this journey, but it's damn near close. You're in a total state of limbo. You get painful tests and terrifying tests (giant needle to the armpit to biopsy my lymph node was my least favorite).

Here's what happened for me: a routine mammogram found calcifications the radiologist didn't like, and so they ordered a second mammogram (which was pretty routine for me—remember my dense breast tissue?). Normally, these are fine. I get the all clear, and I go on my merry way.

Not this year.

This year, they told me I needed a biopsy.

Biopsies can be done any number of ways: in an MRI machine, with the help of an ultrasound, or in a mammogram machine. Mine was done sitting upright, with my face plastered against a mammogram machine, my left boob squashed in it, and needles going straight in a millimeter from my nipple.

A very kind nurse held my hand during this (surprisingly painful process), and then I went home and woke up the next day looking like the Hulk had punched me in the chest, with black and blue knuckle marks to prove it.

That biopsy came back malignant.

Then, I had:

An appointment with a breast surgeon.

An appointment with an oncologist.

A second opinion with a breast surgeon.

A second opinion with another oncologist.

An MRI.

Blood sample for genetic testing to see if cancer is in my genes.

An ultrasound.

A consultation with a plastic surgeon about reconstruction surgery.

Another biopsy (of the lymph node) that involved a needle to the armpit with ultrasound.

Yet another MRI, with the threat of another needle to the armpit, but they couldn't find the mass on the right side they wanted to biopsy—it had naturally been absorbed in my body. It had read the room and was like *I'm not getting stabbed with another fucking armpit needle, thank you very much. I'm... out.*

And all these tests and visits took more than six weeks, just to figure out I was going to have surgery first. Then. . .we'll see.

It was eight full weeks of who-the-hell-knows-what's-happening, hurry-up-and-wait in the Limbo from Hell.

What you will completely lose during this process is your patience.

You will want to punch every single radiologist holding a needle, and every single scheduling nurse that tells you the earliest appointment is in three weeks.

Take a deep breath.

Remember, cancer IS the enemy, and cancer is the one you really want to yell at.

The thing I always kept in mind in this time was: **Measure three times. Cut once.**

I was in a hurry to get treatment, yes, but I didn't want five surgeries when I could just have one. This isn't a craft project, either. This is your body, so wouldn't you want your caregivers to make *damn sure* they know what they're doing before they cut you open?

If they weren't sure about the lymph nodes, they might go in, take one, sew me up, and then decide they needed another one and have to open me up again.

No, thank you.

Measure three times. Cut once.

That made sense to me.

Of course, breast cancer is a messy bitch, so you may measure three times AND cut three times anyway, but at least you've got a shot of having minimum surgery if your doctors take in all the information they can before they cut you open.

Because there could be any number of things that happen during or after surgery that means you'll need another surgery, like an infection or the cancer is bigger than they thought. Or they found it in a lymph node and have to keep going back, taking nodes until one comes back clear, but if you can do everything you can now, to avoid extra surgeries, I mean, doesn't that make sense?

I don't like surgery.

Surgery freaks me out.

If you like anesthesia and having strangers cut on you, then knock yourself out! Measure no times and cut a bazillion!

But, measuring three times and cutting once, this helped me keep things in perspective.

And do you know what else? I needed those two months to get in shape, to get my mind right, to stop bawling uncontrollably in the shower, and to get a handle on my fear (spoiler— the fear overwhelmed me often, and I just had to acknowledge it, pat it on the head while it barked its head off, and then let it wash over me).

The limbo and being a human pin cushion sucked, but it also allowed me time to accept my diagnosis. To get my battle plan together. To have my mini-pity party (several, actually) and then move on. It allowed me the time I needed to choose to be a survivor and not a victim.

Nobody wants to wait.

We want treatment. We want that damn cancer cut out of us forever.

But sometimes, in the wait, there's a gift. I know that feels like spiritual mumbo jumbo, but it's true.

You might need that time. You can also use that time to your advantage to assemble your battle plan. It takes time to put together your training montage.

What the hell is going on? Let's talk about what they're looking for.

Why all the needles, the biopsies, and the tests? Why don't they just cut the damn thing out already?

Well, they're trying to find out how big and bad it is.

I'm not going to get into the science talk at all because you've got a Terrifying Phone Book for that. But I'm going to tell you a story. This is a GENERAL story, not intended to be used as medical fact. Again, I am not a medical professional.

But cancer, as we've discussed, is a Messy Bitch. She's at a bar (that's the inner duct of your breast), and she's with her too-loud friends. She's talking about getting back with her toxic, asshole ex, and everyone in the party has had enough of her, but she's ordering more rounds and is definitely going to fucking call that dude whom everyone hates and probably hook-up with him by night's end. She's screaming at the bartender, "*I'm* not overserved, you're overserved!" and things are about to get messy.

This, my friends, is Stage 0. This is non-invasive, intra-duct, in-situ cancer. She's still at her first bar. She hasn't hopped.

But the bartender kicks her and her noisy friends out on the street. She pukes on the sidewalk. They stumble down the block.

This is what they call invasive Stage One cancer. Caveat: there's stage 1a, and 1b, but we're not going to get that granular, okay? In general, Stage One means they've left the start of the party, and they're out on the street. Cue: being loud and obnoxious, probably falling down, maybe puking at the curb. They are in the breast tissue *outside* the ducts now. This is now invasive cancer because they left the start of the party, and now that messy bitch is trying to make her phone work to call an Uber. She wants to go wherever—anywhere—else because the night is not over until *she* says it's over. The Uber is your lymph node, and if she gets into that fucking Uber, she can go and take her drunken, loud mess anywhere in your body.

This is Stage Two. This is the Uber. If she's gotten the Uber, she could go anywhere: brain, lungs, what have you. But Stage Two means they're just in the lymph node but not found anywhere else.

By Stage Three, they've moved.

Stage Four means they've taken that Uber all over the damn town.

Now, keep in mind, I'm not a medical professional (can you tell by my messy, drunk cancer analogies?). There are all kinds of stages between stages (there's stage 2a, stage 2b, and on and on, that have very specific medical definitions, none of which I covered above). The drunk party story just helped me understand what was happening.

And you probably won't even know for sure WHAT stage you're in until after the surgery, they've grabbed biopsies, and done further lab work on the cancer itself.

There are a whole lot of statistics about your rates of beating every stage of cancer. Just know this: statics are just numbers.

They are not you.

They are not your life.

You are so much more than the odds. You, an individual, can beat those odds. You can crush them. Because you are not the numbers.

You are not the statistics. You are uniquely, amazingly, YOU, and you can make anything possible.

A Man Designed This

The blond nurse in the purple Northwestern Medical shirt is unsure of me because I haven't filled out the paperwork. We are at my first MRI appointment, and we've arrived thirty minutes early as instructed. I thought I had filled out paperwork online—a survey about whether or not I'm claustrophobic, etc. But my answers haven't appeared in My Chart.

We've driven a long way to get this MRI because the MRI machines closer to us were booked up for two months. Sue me if I didn't want to wait that long to figure out what the hell is going on, so I decided to drive an hour to get an earlier appointment.

I want to be extra nice to the tech, so I don't get lodged into a machine with extra contrast in my veins. Then, she tells me I'll have to lay on my stomach, and the props I'll lay on are designed by a man because they're so uncomfortable. This makes me love her immediately.

She shoos me into a dressing room and gives me a litany of instructions that I think I already know: take off any jewelry (check! I didn't even wear my watch today because I didn't want my Apple watch to end up lodged in my sternum when the giant magnets kicked on). She leaves me in what feels like a gym locker room with yet another magenta smock (do they come in any other color?).

I get undressed and put on the gown, extra scared I might have left earrings in that will become magnetized and kill us all, but then remember I never put them in this morning on purpose—I'd left them next to my watch at home. I hesitate on the underwear. Did she tell me just naked from the waist up? Or totally naked?

I used to be so good at listening to instructions, and now I can't even process simple things. I'd been sliding into the white room so often these days, that sometimes I just took ten or twenty second jaunts in there without even realizing it.

I know I have to take off my jeans because of the metal button. But my gray cotton underwear with the newest elastic, which isn't that new? Can I keep those on?

I remember she told me I keep my socks on, which seems like foolish information to retain in my brain, but there it is. The only information I have. Socks on, underwear on too? Or. . . no?

I could shout out, "Hey! What about my underwear?" loud enough for everyone in the waiting room to hear. But I don't. Instead, I just go commando and hope for the best.

I realize my mistake immediately when there's a stepstool with the top step about three and a half feet away from the MRI tray, and the radiologist smiles at me apologetically and says, "You'll just have to kind of launch yourself up here."

Launching bare-ass naked under a thin, scratchy gown feels like a bad combination. Something will go horribly wrong.

It does immediately. I am not a gymnast, and it's immediately obvious when I try to half hop/half slide up on this damn tray. The loose gown does me no good, and I'm flapping out there: butt out, va jay jay singing in the wind. Struggling. Why is this thing so damn high?

The nurse makes a startled sound, and that's when I know for sure she'd said I probably could wear my underwear.

"Let's uh, tuck you in there." She gently folds the gown over me, and I'm immediately worried she thinks I'm a freakish medical nudist who gets my kicks out of startling professionals just trying to do their job.

I need an IV and I get one while I'm busy trying to think in my mind of normal reasons why I wouldn't be wearing underwear, but none of them sound great: I came not wearing any! They got stained! (EW!) They were so old; they disintegrated the second my jeans hit the floor!

Whatever. It's probably not the worst thing she's seen. And now, I'm face down on the damn thing, three inches between me and a towel and so I can't see her expression, which is probably a good thing.

She asks if I want music or not, but she adds about five warnings to having music: it's loud, it cuts in and out, sometimes it's too soft, sometimes it's too loud, she thinks it's annoying, but I'm free to have it.

"The MRI machine does use radio waves, so it interferes with the music," she tells me.

I also suddenly worry that I'll be stuck listening to Barry Manilow the whole time. Now is no time to think about "Copa Cabana".

"I'll take the earplugs," I say, and she helps me put them in, but as all foam earplugs do, they keep popping out. "Actually, I don't think they'll stay in. Maybe I do need earphones?"

"How about just noise cancelling?"

"Great!"

She sets the noise cancelling earphones on my head. And places a bulb attached to a wire to my right hand. Squeeze it if I want to communicate. Don't forget: be still. If I move, I ruin everything.

The tray moves, and I head, feet first/backward into the tube.

I'm not claustrophobic, but being in an MRI machine makes me think for the first time that claustrophobia is a good, solid, reasonable option. I've never panic-meditated so hard in all my life.

Then, the technician turns on the machine, and it sounds like Michael Meyers is on the other side of the tube with a ball pin hammer, and he's also blaring the baseline from the Bee Gees at the same time. I am imagining music where the is none.

Click, click, click. Whirl. Bang, bang, Staying Alive, Staying Alive! Bang, bang, bang, zzzzzzzzzzt!

Just focus on my breathing. Count those breaths. Inhale 1, Inhale 2. I am not stuck in a tube face down. I can't move or the radiologist will be mad and make me stay in here longer. Michael Meyers is not trying to kill me. This machine isn't a monster that will eat me alive.

Sounds like it though.

Bang! Bang! Thunka thunka thunka thuaka. Now it's... *Hey, Now, You're an All Star, get your came on, go play. Bang! Bang!! Zffffffft. Click click. Clack. Bwwweeeep! Bweeeep!* Car alarm! Car alarm! Car alarm! Smoke detector! Smoke Detector!

Bee booo, bee, boo! European Ambulance! European Ambulance!

Bweeep. Bweeeep. Car Alarm again.

One fucking inhale. One fucking exhale. Two. Three. Four. Five.

It's so damn loud. Maybe "Copa Cobana" would've been better than this.

That's some kind of kink.
Afterward, on the drive home, I tell my husband about going commando for the MRI, and he laughs so hard I think he might crash the car.

"I was worried the techs thought flashing them is some kink," I admit.

PJ snorts. "That's a very, very odd kink. I mean, that has not shown up on Pornhub. And, I mean, I've carefully looked through all of it. For science."

"Just doing your part for sociology?"

"Exactly."

How much time do I really have before I definitely need to get this cut out of me?
It depends. There are a lot of metrics about positive outcomes for treatment. Some cancers (like mine) show that eight weeks from diagnosis to surgery (if surgery is the right course of

action first—before chemo) is best. But there are a lot of factors about when to get what treatment and what may raise mortality rates.

There has been a whole lot of research about breast cancer (though there needs to be a whole lot more). Some tumors grow faster than others. One study found in the average wait time between diagnosis and surgery was 31 days, with a range of 8 to 78 days, and in that time the growth rate of different tumors varied quite a bit.

- **Triple-negative tumors:** 1.003 percent growth each day
- **HER2 positive tumors:** 0.850 percent growth each day
- **Luminal B/A tumors (estrogen receptor positive tumors):** 0.208/0.175 percent growth each day[10]

I had HER2 positive cancer, which is not the most common kind of cancer, but it's also more aggressive than Luminal B/A tumors), but you could have a different kind of cancer. And—because cancer is a messy bitch—it's even possible to have multiple different kinds of breast cancer at the same time (oh, yes, it happens).

Don't stress about time passing, but at the same time, don't throw up extra roadblocks yourself.
Clear your calendar so that you can get to the soonest appointment. Cancer is the most important thing on your schedule right now.

---

[10] Lynne Eldridge, MD, "How Long Can You Wait to Have Treatment for Breast Cancer? Delays in Surgery or Chemotherapy and Effects on Survival," *Very Well Health*, March 10, 2024.

Don't have insurance? Are you waiting three months for the enrollment period to kick in?

Don't.

Just... don't.

Skip ahead to Chapter Fourteen: Avoid Soul-Crushing Debt, but also know this: bankruptcy sounds horrible and terrible, but you know what's worse? Waiting three months and moving from Stage 1 to Stage 2 or even—3. Would you rather be poor or would you rather be dead?

Keep the ball moving. That's all.

But delaying feels good because then I can snuggle up in denial and pretend nothing is wrong. Do I really want to know?

There will be days when you want to stick your head in the sand and pretend everything is fine, and the last thing you want to do is pick up the phone when your nurse navigator calls.

I'm with you. Burying your head in the sand is cozy and nice, and who doesn't love a day at the beach? Is there an all-inclusive resort there with a swim-up bar? Count me in.

But, my friend, knowledge will be your friend. Facing the thing—however bad it is—will be better than ignoring it.

Why?

Because once you drag that horrible monster out from under your bed and into the light, the monster isn't so scary anymore.

Take any creepy movie ever. When you can't see the monster, your imagination runs wild, and you start to think the thing is scarier than it is because you can't see it. Once you lay eyes on it, once you understand it, it becomes less scary.

It's still terrifying, don't get me wrong.

But you take away some of its power when you understand what it is you're really dealing with.

And you won't know how to fight it unless you find out what it is.

So, take the millionth needle poke, or the third MRI, or the umpteenth blood test. Figure out what you're dealing with so you can fight it with all you've got.

The length between tests is killing me faster than the cancer. The long wait times (days, sometimes even weeks) before you can get that next phase of your testing (biopsy, MRI, etc.) scheduled can be a unique kind of torture all on its own. Despite the clear urgency on your part (I've got freakin' cancer!), sometimes it might feel like your medical team is taking their sweet-ass time figuring out a plan of action. Now, some wait is expected, but too long a wait isn't okay (and we'll talk about medical teams more in Chapter Seven: Not a\All Doctors Are Good).

Also the speed at which you get care, and the level of that care will depend on where you live and the resources available near you. People who live near big city centers with large medical groups are likely to have better care than those in rural areas, and they're more likely to have their cancer caught in earlier stages. While about 16% of the U.S. population lives in rural areas, only 3% of oncologists practice there.[11]

I lived in the suburbs of Chicago, near all kinds of medical facilities, and I still found myself looking at long wait times for some tests. I asked about other locations in my medical network that I could drive to, that might have a sooner MRI open, or ultrasound available, and often, I did get earlier appointments (even if I had to drive an hour to get one).

---

[11] "Rural-Urban Disparities in Cancer," Cancer Map Stories, Gis.Cancer.gov., Nov 7, 2024.

Do not be afraid to raise your hand and ask for options. Think outside the box. Does your sister live in a place with better doctors?

Don't assume the best options are near you because they might not be.

Get used to raising your hand, too, because you are going to need to be your own best advocate for care.

It's just like a bee sting. In your armpit.

The doctor maneuvers the ultrasound wand around my left armpit, digging hard to find the right lymph node. This is the biopsy I've been dreading for the last week. DREADing.

I didn't exactly love the first biopsy. What for the click CLACK—SLAM BAM, NEEDLE TO THE NIPPLE, NO THANK YOU, MA'AM!!

I'm staring up at the small rectangular picture in the ceiling, between the regular tiles, the picture of the cherry blossom tree, a random shrub, and blue skies. I guess it's better than a picture of hellfire, or an incoming missile, or a tornado. It's supposed to be relaxing and comforting, even though none of this is going to be comfortable. The picture can't fool me. I'm not here to picnic in a beautiful park in Japan, okay?

A) Biopsies aren't fun. A needle into your body with a small tube that sucks things out isn't fun for anyone.

B) I'm going to have to wait three to four days to see if the cancer has gotten into that Uber and headed to a third or fourth bar. That messy bitch has just begun her night, and if she's escaped to a new bar, which will mean chemo first, surgery later.

C) The lidocaine they use might as well be baby aspirin. Seriously. They never give me enough. I may be small, but my tolerance for drugs is high, people.

The radiologist is nice. His voice is gentle. He reminds me of a grade schoolteacher or a librarian. Gentle and kind.

"We're just going to go over a few more things before we begin," he tells me.

"Are you allergic to any medicines?" the nurse asks me.

"No. Just cats," I joke. "As long as we aren't sneaking them into the exam room, I should be good."

"Okay, and… do we have the marker?" the doctor asks the nurse. "Did we check with the surgeon about which marker?"

"I'll go check," the nurse says and leaves the room.

The marker is a tiny piece of metal, too small to set off a metal detector but large enough for a surgeon to find so that she knows which lymph node to grab. I've since learned there are all kinds of markers. Some are like a radio beacon, which set off a sound until they're located.

"Did she want the one that beeps? I just don't want to be a smoke detector with low batteries," I joke.

He laughs a little. "Is that the one she wanted?"

"I don't know. The nurse navigator told me there were a lot of different kinds, and I don't know, that's the one I remember. But I bet you know more than me."

I hope you know more than me.

The nurse is back. She says the name of the marker (I don't know what it means), but it's not the beeping one.

"We're going to give you some lidocaine to numb the area," he says, and I try not to sigh because I already know lidocaine gives as much punch as half a baby Tylenol. "You'll feel a little sting here. Just like a bee. Just stay still a minute."

There is a prick, as I lie, arm flung over the top of my head, and I wonder: Who on earth holds still for a bee sting? In the armpit?

I am not properly doing my job as a human protecting my body if I let a *bee* sting my *armpit*. Windmill arms should've properly gotten rid of that little fella *way* before he got anywhere close to my armpit. Hand? Sure. Arm. Probably. But armpit? I would die first.

I'm just saying, the metaphor might need work. Instead of bee sting, how about a little fingernail prick? How about a little pinch (maybe from an angel)? Or, how about, this is just gonna suck for a minute. Wait it out.

But, I lie still as the burning sensation of lidocaine beneath the skin sets in. I wait.

"Can you feel it when I touch you?" There's a finger to the armpit now.

"Not really." I'm kind of shocked how well *his* lidocaine is working where the others failed. Did the other radiologists even give me any?

I'm pretty sure he's making the incision. They have to cut you before they stick the needle/tube/suction thingy inside. He spends some time getting the tube into place. I wait, arm above my head.

"You're going to here a clicking sound. In three, two. . .one." *CLICK CLACK!* It sounds like a staple gun. It feels like one too.

I remember the sound from the last biopsy that stabbed my nipple. I might have a PTSD flashback. I jump. It's a loud sound, but more than that, there's a sharp pain afterward.

"Is that painful?" he asks me because I've jumped out of my skin.

"Yes, a little sharp," I admit.

"More lidocaine," he says immediately, and I begin to like him more right then. "It's really just like Novocain but for your body."

"Too bad you don't have laughing gas," I say and I'm not joking. Laughing gas would make this awesome instead of terrible.

"That's actually pretty bad for you," he tells me.

"I think what you mean is way more fun for me," I say, and he laughs a little. The nurse laughs more. I might use jokes as shields for any occasion: social anxiety, nervousness, getting my armpit stung by a bee.

"Okay, you're going to here that click in three again. Three, two. . . one!" *CLICK CLACK.* This time, it's just a loud noise. I don't feel like I'm begin stapled from the inside.

"That's better," I tell them.

"Good," the nurse says.

"We've gotten one sample, but we usually get three or four."

He click-clacks me seven more times.

But he's got the lidocaine way up, so I don't care so much. It's a gentle push to the armpit. But the click-clack is still unnerving. I have the sudden urge to tell about a hundred more jokes to feel more comfortable. If you can't tell by now, I crack jokes when I'm nervous.

"Okay," he says finally. "We've got the samples. Now, I'll just put the marker in."

"There!" he says after a moment. "All done. You did great."

"Phew, I'm glad because I'm ridiculously ticklish and I was worried."

This gets a genuine laugh from both doctor and nurse.

The doctor leaves and the nurse applies pressure to my armpit. There's nothing like a causal conversation when a stranger is pinching a bleeder while you're half naked, one boob out, one arm over your head. Naturally, we talk about the weather.

"It's gotten to be perfect fall weather," she exclaims, and I agree. Hey, we're in Chicago, so when we get sixty-degree days they are to be celebrated. We have two seasons: winter and July. So, it's either ninety degrees, or it's negative twenty. Sixty is something to celebrate. We talk about the weather for what seems like hours, and then we transition to people endlessly coughing. The conversation stretches on for hours, but it's probably just ten minutes.

She releases the pressure. "Okay! Good, I think you've stopped."

Yeah, for me and my clotting cells. Yeah.

The clock is ticking.

Whether or not your medical team finds this testing stage urgent, keep in mind that the best outcomes typically are starting some kind of treatment relatively soon after diagnosis. My surgeon did want to measure three times, but she was also very aware the clock was ticking. Once it was determined that I would have surgery first, then she scheduled it on the date eight weeks to the day of my diagnosis, just in the nick of time.

It's okay to ask—and continue to ask—where you are on that timeline and share your concern about how quickly the testing is going.

Also, you're in charge of your care. Make sure you ask as many questions as you need (I'll keep repeating this again and again) to understand why you need a certain test, what they're hoping (or not hoping) to find, and to be fully informed at every stage.

Remember, this too, will pass.

For many women, this not knowing, this constant ping-pong of tests, is the worst part. It's the worst part because you don't know how bad the cancer is, and you don't know what your options are to fight it.

Once you know, things will be calmer. Better. More certain. It's the uncertainty in these first few weeks or even months that are the real torture.

You WILL get to certain. You WILL figure out how bad the cancer is, and you WILL get a slate of options to choose from, including what the hell you're going to do about it.

Remember this is the crappy time. This is the scary time. The time you're so distracted you forget to wear underwear in the MRI machine.

You can't see the monster under your bed because it's hiding, but when it comes out in the light, hopefully, it won't be as bad as you fear.

You won't always be a human pin cushion.

This, too, shall pass.

Pep talk #3:

Hey, Soldier. Getting tired of people stabbing you with needles? I know. I've been there.

"When will this fucking end?" you shout into the universe. "I just want the answers already."

You'll get them. You will. Now is the time for you to dig deep inside you for the patience none of us really have.

While you do this, I want to congratulate you—for NOT sticking your head in the sand, for doing the hard things (and they are so fucking hard) to get the answers you need so you understand what treatments are best.

This is YOU being the adult in your life. This is YOU being strong. You thought you were afraid and weak? Hell, no. This phase of pokes and prodding and being on hold to make an appointment shows just what a kick-ass warrior you are.

So, keep going. One step at a time. One battle at a time.

That's how you win the war.

Chapter Four

Breaking the News—Brace Yourself for the Pity and Pivot

"Bad news travels fast. Good news takes the scenic route."

—Doug Larson

"Mom? What is it? What's wrong?" my youngest daughter asks me, all nerves, as she climbs into the front seat of our Mazda SUV as I pick her up from cross country practice. She knows I had a biopsy, and we're awaiting results. Also, unbeknownst to me then, she took one look at my puffy, red eyes and immediately gleaned the news wasn't good. "Is it the biopsy? Did you get the results?"

The anxiousness in her voice breaks my heart. It breaks my heart because I know that instead of being able to comfort her, to tell her everything will be all right, I have to tell her everything isn't all right. It's far from fucking all right.

It's cancer.

I planned to drive the six minutes home and tell her there, but she can't wait. She wants to know now. I pull into the small parking lot of the park next to the school, and I have her full, undivided attention. I look at her and see the little girl who lit up at the sight of her Dora the Explorer birthday cake. I see the toddler, not even two, who declared she was done with diapers—and miraculously, was. I see the whip smart teenager she is now—always quick with a quip, a champion arguer, loyal to a fault to those she loves, the first to jump in and argue against any punishment—either for herself or her siblings. She's such a fantastic debater that she'd make an excellent defense attorney, and on more than one occasion, I pleaded with her to stop arguing with me and just make plans to go to law school. She'd argue so logically and relentlessly that as much as I hated to admit it, if we ever debated a house rule, nine times out of ten I lost the debate, and would have to retreat to the "Because I'm the mom and I said so" closing argument—weak at best.

"The biopsy came back, and... it's cancer," I say, as tears immediately well in her eyes, and I think about how I'd feel if I were fifteen and my mom told me she had breast cancer—and panic chokes me. "But it's caught early, so I'm going to be fine, really—I will be fine."

But even I don't believe the words coming out of my mouth because, sure, that's what the doctors said, but there was a whole marathon between now and fine. I had no idea, actually that I'd really be fine, and my daughter always could read between the lines. She's crying now.

"I'm sorry," I say. "I'm so sorry." And I was—because parents of teenagers aren't supposed to have cancer. They're not supposed to suck the drama out of the room. They're supposed to let teens have the main stage with their on-time angst.

Parents should be the calm, boring voices of reason. Parents don't get sick—they're not allowed to get sick even when they are. I felt on all levels that I was failing her. I was making her grow up too fast. Making her be the caretaker when this was something she shouldn't have to worry about until she's oh so much older.

"Why are you sorry?" she sobs. "You've got *cancer*."

Delivering the Shit Sandwich No One Ordered

The thing about telling people this news is that it's an atomic bomb in people's days. The closer you are to the person you tell, the worse this news is.

The atomic bomb of news in your back pocket will hurt those closest to you the most. It will leave them speechless. It will bring tears. It will bring to life that fear you've been battling every minute since your diagnosis—that this is as bad as you thought.

Nobody likes bad news.

In fact, people will go to great lengths to avoid bad news.

"Ignorance is bliss" is a real thing—most people avoid bad news when they can. Most people avoid checking their 401k balances after a dip in stock prices for fear of getting bad news,[12] and a whopping 90% of people said they'd prefer NOT to know the date of their death.[13]

Take those who have a higher risk of developing Huntington's Disease, a terrible neurogenerative disorder, that's incurable. Healthcare providers can offer a blood DNA test to see whether high-risk patients (those whose parents had Huntington's Disease) will develop the condition in their lifetime. Keep in mind that an early diagnosis wouldn't affect the outcome as the disease is incurable, but knowing about it definitely affected major life decisions of those who suffer from it. For instance, if you knew you had it, you might choose not to have biological children, since you could pass the gene on to them. Or, you might choose to retire early so you could enjoy more of your life before the disease set in.

---

[12] Nachum Sicherman, George Loewenstein, Duane J. Seppi, Stephen P. Utkus, "Financial Attention," *The Review of Financial Studies*, November 19, 2015.

[13] Gigerenzer, G., & Garcia-Retamero, R., "Cassandra's regret: The psychology of not wanting to know," *Psychological Review*, 2017.

Despite this, research shows a whopping 93% of the high-risk population choose NOT to get the blood test and avoid possible bad news.[14] Even more surprising, untested people with a high risk of developing Huntington's tended to convince themselves they were totally fine, and not at risk. They were blindingly optimistic, and greatly underestimated the chances of developing the disease.[15] I mean, if you're going to go in for denial, go *all in* for denial. I get it. I'd be the same way.

Another fascinating part about bad news is that, while most of us avoid it, we do pay attention to bad news more than good news.[16] It makes sense because we're programmed to listen to bad news for survival. If someone in our tribe warned us about poisonous mushrooms, we'd probably pay more attention than if they told us about harmless flowers growing in a field. At least, those of us who survived would've paid more attention. Those who didn't prioritize bad news would just forget, go pick the flowers, then devour the mushrooms, and perish.

Now you, yourself, may have been avoiding your own bad news about cancer, and now that it's your turn to share bad news with relatives, friends, and colleagues, you may feel hesitant to do so. You might not want to blow up their days.

Some cancer patients opt to keep cancer a secret from their families and those closest to them because they're so afraid of unleashing the nuclear bomb of bad news. Or they want to suffer in silence (if you're leaning this way, please read Chapter

---

[14] Eva M. Krockow Ph.D, "Ignorance Is Bliss: Why People Avoid Bad News," *Psychology Today*, July 9, 2020.

[15] Emily Oster, Ira Shoulson, E. Ray Dorsey. "Optimal Expectations and Limited Medical Testing: Evidence from Huntington Disease," *American Economic Review*, April 2013.

[16] Hara Estroff Marano, "Why We Love Bad News," *Psychology Today*, May 23, 2003.

Five: Martyrs Die Alone). You might be tempted to do this because telling people makes it real and you can't have it be real.

I get this. I do.

But you will need to share this. It will be hard. It will be horrible but tell the people closest to you. Tell your kids and your spouse, whomever is closest in your orbit. Do not keep this a secret from them. Do not put on a brave face and NOT tell your grown son.

The people closest to you will be most affected, but if you keep this a secret, they WILL be furious with you. And for good reason.

Swap places with them. If your spouse had this horrible thing happening and they didn't tell you, how would YOU feel? If your grown children kept cancer a secret from you because they "didn't want to be a bother," or "didn't want to scare you," how would YOU feel? Furious. Betrayed. Helpless.

You'd feel like they deliberately left you out of a life-altering, potentially life-taking, diagnosis and refused to even let you help. You'd think back on all those months when they were suffering, wishing you could've done something—even if it was just sending a damn lavender candle.

So, as hard as this is, TELL those closest to you.

But you get to decide who to tell, when to tell them, and how.
I decided I wanted to let individuals know before I posted anything to social media, lest people feel left out or something dumb like that (believe me, people do take offense), but every single time I told someone, it got more real and more terrifying.

The more people you tell, the more real this shit becomes.

I found myself not even believing my own diagnosis on some days, but the more times I said, "I've got breast cancer," the more reality sunk in. Shit. I've got *breast cancer.* Sometimes, I'll be honest, I felt as horrible and shocked as the people I was telling.

It's terrifying, but that's okay. You need to tell people because you're going to need people to help you.

Just tell people at your own pace. Some might prefer to tell everyone at once, but I found that exhausting. I told a few people daily over about a week's time. I told some people in person, some by phone, and some by text, and then I eventually posted something online. I went at my own pace. Figure out the pace that works for you and do it.

Also, you will be asked all the questions you can't answer but wish you could. What's the treatment plan? What stage is it? What's the prognosis? Will you need surgery? When? Chemo? Radiation? Do you know what stage it is yet?

No, you don't know. You wish you did, but you don't.

Explaining all you don't know about your cancer, again and again, can be exhausting.

The worst thing is you get to tell yourself this shitty news every morning.

During the early days, I woke up and I didn't remember right away that I had cancer. In that twilight of reaching for the alarm, it felt like every other day.

And then I remembered.

Oh, shit. I had breast cancer.

This sucks.

This happened every single time I woke up. I got clobbered with a pile of bricks.

Every.

Single.

Morning.

And it didn't matter when I woke up either. It could be 2 am, or 7 am, there would be that pile of bricks waiting for me.

Bam. Hi there. It's cancer. Thought you'd dream me away? Oh, no. I'm still here.

Stupid bitch. I really, seriously, hate her.

So, you get to tell yourself this news too, every day.

That means, you get a break about who you tell. If you want to be "normal" for as long as you can, listen, sister, I'm not judging you.

The one thing I want you to know now is that I'm never judging you. Whether you tell people or not, whether you follow any advice in this book or not, whether you get treatment or not, only you can walk your path. No one else can do it for you. You are the one that has to fight this battle/climb this mountain in flipflops, so YOU get to decide.

Nobody will say the right thing and that's okay.

When you break this news, nobody will say the right thing because, really, there is no right thing to say. I mean, the best thing I could think of to hear would be, "Oh? You've got breast cancer? Well, what a coincidence, I just invented a cure. I've got it right here in my back pocket. . . "

You'll get a lot of *I'm so sorry*, of course, and a lot of people who rush to ask about the next steps or treatment, which you don't know because you're in Human Pincushion Mode. Personally, some people asked immediately if cancer ran in my family.

It doesn't.

Some people will say the WORST things. Like, "Everything happens for a reason" or "God wouldn't give you anything you can't handle."

Please, if anyone tells you this, let me be the first one to get in line to punch them in the face.

As you might already have guessed, these not-so-truisms are dismissive and wildly untrue. You are human. This shit is hard. It's not something anyone is "meant" to handle, it's something we all have to solider through, teeth gritted and fists balled.

Also, sometimes, you go through something absolutely terrible, and it never makes sense.

People say these stupid things because they don't have anything else to say, and they heard this once, or someone told it to *them*, so they are just passing along shitty one-liners to you. And if you're like me, you might realize you yourself have said the same dumb things to people with bad news because you didn't know what else to say.

People handle bad news differently, and they handle scary news in even more creative ways.

Some people want to drop everything and help you (these are the keepers of course. I'll talk about The Helpers in a minute. They are the GEMS of life). Other people want to know what *you* did wrong (Having shitty genes! Wearing aluminum deodorant! Eating too much sugar! Drinking too much!). They want to know this so they can reassure themselves *they* won't get it. These people might be assholes, or they might just be scared.

People get scared. You—their friend/relative/coworker/classmate—might be the first time they've gotten so close to breast cancer, and their first instinct will be to put it in a box that can't hurt them. Again, remember how we pay attention to bad news more than good for our own survival? They're just desperately trying to key in relative facts into their brains so they themselves can avoid harm later.

If cancer runs in your family, or if you mainlined weed killer, then they don't have to worry about getting it *themselves*. Here's the thing—no one knows the cause of most breast cancer diagnoses. Only about a quarter of cases are genetic.[17] The other three-fourths? Who the hell knows? You probably

---

[17] "About Breast Cancer," The National Human Genome Research Institute, November 2014.

won't because, most of the time, there is no rhyme or reason about why someone gets cancer. And you'll probably never know.

People will ask you a lot of questions. It's okay to simply say, "I don't want to talk about that," or even give them a white lie, "I don't know," even if you do. Remember, you can tell them as much or as little about your situation as you deem fit. You don't have to answer all fifty questions. You don't have to answer any at all.

Some people will tell you to be a fighter.
Some others will prop you up and tell you that you're a fighter and that you've got this. While they mean well, it might feel dismissive. I seriously got into the mode where I wanted to punch anyone who told me this straight in the face.

They meant well. I know they did.

But it felt like a dismissive shrug. "Oh, you've got to battle Goliath with a little slingshot? You got this."

Seriously, though? Have you seen my wimpy arms? I've never been able to do an unassisted pull-up in my entire life.

When people told me I'm a fighter, I instantly thought: no, I'm not.

I'm a pacifist.

I've never been in a fistfight in my life, and I hope to die never having been in one. I hate conflict. I avoid conflict so much I stayed in the wrong marriage for a decade because I didn't want to mention that I was unhappy and maybe I'd made a mistake. I will go to great lengths to avoid an argument (probably why the first marriage didn't last—I've gone to therapy and worked on this). I will even listen to people I am totally opposed to—politically, religiously, any kind of -ly— and rather than argue with them, I'll just try to keep my face from betraying absolute horror. Chances are, I don't even say a word to dislodge someone from trying to convince me the world is flat.

Fighter? Me? I mean, I'm sarcastic sometimes. Does that count?

I'm not ready. I'm not a fighter. I've never been a fighter. I can't do this.

Also, I think the "you're a fighter" moniker is fundamentally unfair. When they tell you to fight cancer, they're basically telling you that it's just all ON YOU to defeat it. Nobody does this with other kinds of ailments. No one tells you to kick pneumonia with a reverse roundhouse. Nobody expects anybody to put a sleeper hold on diabetes. Can you imagine if we told people that all you had to do was give heart disease a good upper cut?

"You got high blood pressure? Guess it's time for you to hit the dojo. Cholesterol is gonna get his ass HANDED to him."

No. With all those other things, we just rely on medicine and medical professionals to do their job. Antibiotics. Insulin. Blood pressure meds. There's no added call to action, except maybe change your diet and exercise. Or avoid salt or sugar.

Yet, somehow, cancer is different. Somehow, it's all in our control to beat it if we just "fight" it somehow, even though it's hidden, deep within our bodies, somewhere we can't reach or even see. I'm just supposed to get my Batman cancer-fighting suit and go vigilante the shit out of it. I'm supposed to suddenly be a John Wick assassin taking my revenge? I hate guns and I'm terribly uncoordinated.

People mean well. They're giving you a compliment. They're telling you that you're tough. But I didn't feel tough. I felt scared. I saw the bat signal in the sky, but I didn't want to answer it. I wanted to hide in my bat cave, eat ice cream by the pint, and let a qualified medical professional handle it— someone smarter and better trained than me.

Other people will simply say "you've got this" which is another variation on "you're a fighter." The sentiment is sweet, but it rings hollow because I don't feel like I DO have this at all.

My retirement planning isn't even on track, and my credit card debt is too large. I'm terrible at dieting. Worse at adhering to Dry January. I don't fold my clothes right. It's not just fitted sheets, but it's *everything*. I wad T-shirts in a ball and throw them in my drawer and hope they won't come out too wrinkled—but I've "got" cancer?! I mean, WTF? Do you even know me?

Sigh.

Other people will be more in denial than you are.

There are yet others who'll be in denial about the whole thing—worse than you are—and who will skip right on over to the end: *You'll be fine. They caught it early/kind of early/I mean you're not dead yet, right? They've got all kinds of treatments and you'll be fine. Phew. Aren't you glad you'll be fine?*

Except you're not fucking fine.

I know.

I see you.

Nobody with this diagnosis is fine (see Chapter One: Your New Normal, Also This Normal Fucking Sucks).

And the "you'll be fine" dismissal also runs roughshod over the fact that all those treatments are horrible and nothing happens overnight. Oh, I'll just get chemo, my hair and fingernails will fall out, and I don't feel like eating anything ever? Oh, sure. I'm FINE. So fucking fine! Ha. What a walk in the park. So glad I've got nothing to worry about.

Everyone will know someone who's been through it.

Keep in mind that every woman's experience is different. There is no one-size-fits-all for this shitty ride, so even if you do talk to someone else, remember that their experience might not be your experience. As we talked about in Chapter One, this is your own unique nightmare. Congrats!

Some of those people might not align with your beliefs. Maybe they're too into traditional treatment, or they're not into traditional treatment enough. Maybe they swear by fava beans as the cure-all. Whatever it is, take it with a grain of salt.

Talk to them.

Don't.

They might be in the sisterhood, and they might be your new best friend, but they also don't have to be.

The worst of all? The pity and pivot.

Most people you'll tell will be rightly horrified that you've got cancer.

At the same time, a big block of people will be shocked and stunned, doing what most people do when they hear the scary, horrible news of breast cancer.

You get what I call the **pity and pivot**.

This is how it works: *Oh, my gosh, I'm so sorry to hear that. Wow. Horrible. How are you holding up? Um-hm. Well, I'm so glad they caught it early. Gosh. That's got to be hard. Um-hm. Pause. Did you hear about Riley's divorce? Her husband ran off with a woman he met at a business conference. I am not kidding!*

Pity. Then, pivot.

Nobody wants to marinate in bad news, and scary news is, well, scary. Remember how most people will go to great lengths to avoid bad news? So, most people want to give you the pity and pivot. I mean if *you* could pivot away from this news, you would, but you can't.

You have to wake up with it, shower with it, eat with it, work with it, and can't ever fucking leave it for one fucking minute, but these other people, on the outside, they hear it for five minutes and want to run away. And I can't blame them. I'd want to run away, too.

So some people will just give you what they can give you. And these same people will ask how you are later, and then quickly steer the conversation elsewhere.

They do this because they're uncomfortable and they're afraid. For you. For themselves. You have to stare death straight in the face. They've told you death exists when they've been blithely living their lives wrapped up in a cocoon of denial.

Remember how you were there just a little while ago, before the diagnosis? Later, these same people will tell you how brave you are, and you will know in your core JUST how brave because you never pitied and pivoted. You couldn't pivot. You had to stare Death straight in the face. You didn't look away. You didn't run from the bad news. You lived it. Every day of your treatment.

A few people will get it right.
One of my closest friends actually did say the perfect thing when I told her I had cancer. She told me to take the time I needed for myself, and that this was the time to be selfish (oh, she was definitely right about that), that all my (real) friends would understand.

She said that diagnosis day was a marker in my life, that I'd come to see it as Before that Day and After that Day, and the experience would change me. She was right. She told me to take every day forward one day at a time. Because that's all we can do. One day at a time.

Don't go taking on everything right now. Just take on today.
And I'll tell you something else: when you battle through this and you emerge as a survivor, which you will, because I'm rooting for you and because you'll dig deep in yourself and find a reserve you never even knew was there, you will be stronger than you were before. I promise you. You will. You might not feel like it now, but you will be.

You'll take every day one at a time. As a Human Pincushion and worse, you'll get stronger. Every day. Just a little bit. Even on your super weak days, you'll be getting stronger.

Yes, you'll get the pity and pivots, but you'll get stronger because you find you don't need platitudes from friends who maybe aren't the rocks you thought they were. You'll find the people in your life who don't pivot, who stare at the ugly, scary things with you, and those will be your Helpers. You'll have the people who don't forget you, who just keep checking with the "How are you?" even though asking that question is scary AF for them because they might get the bad news that other people strenuously avoid. And that simple text can make you feel seen and loved, at a time when you need it the most. You might get a lot of meals delivered to your door, or a lot of flowers, or a lot of surprising gifts like socks that say: "If you can read this, I'm kicking cancer's ass" or "Cancer picked the wrong bitch." Oh, did she ever.

People don't always say the right things, but most people *do* the right things.

Look for The Helpers

The one thing that most people do say when you break the news is: "Let me know if there's anything I can do to help."

Most people mean it, too. Cancer is the kind of bad news that turns most everyone into Helpers.

When terrorists crashed planes into the World Trade Center on 9/11, the entire country was in shock. I was in shock. I was in my late twenties, unaware that there were people in the world who hated Americans so badly they'd kill themselves to kill us.

In processing that horrible day and moment, I remember that, at that time, Mr. Rogers, the creator of *Mr. Rogers' Neighborhood*, recorded encouraging videos, helping us to cope.

One of his most famous quotes was: "When I was a boy and I would see scary things in the news, my mother would say to me, 'Look for The Helpers. You will always find people who are helping.'"

It's easy to see all the downsides to cancer and to rage against it, but don't forget to look for The Helpers. They're there.

I've had so many, and I'm so grateful for them.

The very kind and chatty nurse who held my hand during the painful biopsy. The knowledgeable surgeon who told it to me straight and didn't sugarcoat anything. The geneticist. The physical therapist. The health insurance agent who helped get me covered as my COBRA was running out. The financial planner. My counselor reminded me of times when I'd been strong before and that challenge was nothing new to me. My friends, my amazing friends, who texted and checked on me, who made clear I could talk as much or as little about what was going on, who celebrated me when I showed up to dinner and when I was too tired and worn out to come. Who let me know I was never forgotten. I was on their minds. My family, parents, and kids. My amazing husband cancelled fishing trips, barbeque competitions, work trips, and meetings to be by my side for all the appointments.

Because, like he always says, you are what you do when it counts.

I'm not religious, but I am spiritual, and I do believe in angels. People who carry in them a divinity, who lift you up when you need it, who share their light with you when yours grows dim.

What I realize now more than ever is that what you do in your life, how you show up for other people, affects how they show up for you. Also, the kind of people you let have real estate in your life is important, too.

I had plenty of toxic people that I said "no" to: bad friends, ex-boyfriends, ex-fiancés—people who would not be up for this moment. People not sturdy enough to lean on. People who would fold like a house of cards. I'm so grateful that I told them "no" many years ago, that I took on the heartache, and the tears, and the pain back then—so that they weren't in my life now. So that now I only have Helpers.

These Helpers are strong. These Helpers I can lean on. I'm not afraid they'll fold.

Pep talk #4:

Hey, sister. This is one of the hardest parts, breaking bad news to those you love and care about. It's even harder when you feel like that news is brushed aside or dismissed. People don't mean to be assholes. Sometimes, they just aren't equipped to handle terrifying news, and they say dumb things. This is okay. People don't have to say the right thing, and you'll find the true Helpers in your life. These people will be your rock in hard times.

Don't feel bad for dropping the atomic bomb of bad news. Right now, it feels like ALL bad news, but you WILL have good news. You will. And when you deliver that to your family and friends, they will celebrate right along with you. Times are dark now, but the sun WILL rise. And imagine how excited you will be to share the GOOD news when it comes!

Keep on going. It won't be bad news forever.

Chapter Five

Martyrs Die Alone. Don't Be A Martyr. Nobody Gets Bonus Points for Suffering in Silence.

"Cancer is a journey, but you walk the road alone. There are many places to stop along the way and get nourishment—you just have to be willing to take it."

—Emily Hollenberg

Some people will want to try to white knuckle this themselves, tell people who offer help, "No, thanks, I've got it" when they don't and refuse to let their kids/husband/wife/sister help them even when they're offering ALL THE TIME.

And who can blame us?

We're taught basically from the time we can walk that we're supposed to do EVERYTHING and we're never supposed to complain. We're always supposed to be grateful and, for fuck's sake, no matter what kind of terrible day you've had or the fact you've got CANCER, definitely always SMILE to perfect strangers. Otherwise, you're a bitch or you're a problem or you're hard to work with.

And we're just innately supposed to know how to be the best parents and spouses, and if you ask for help, then maybe you don't know what you're doing and everyone will point and laugh and criticize you to fucking death. We all know we can't win, no matter how hard we work, how much we love our kids, how much we prepare for meetings, or how little we eat. So, for goodness' sake, never, ever ask for any help with anything and only ever post perfect pictures of you on all your socials.

I think, deep down, you know this is bullshit.

Cancer is the perfect excuse to call bullshit on bullshit.

Everybody needs help dealing with cancer.

And while people might still criticize your choices (they're the assholes, FYI), you'll still need help on the journey.

Time for some hard truths: nobody gets a special medal for going to doctor's appointments alone.

Nobody gets a badge of honor for getting stuffed into an MRI tube with NO ONE waiting for them to take them through a drive-thru for a stack of hot fries and a chocolate shake—just because.

Nobody gets a ribbon for not complaining.

You might feel that you're taking on extra responsibility so that your family doesn't have to suffer, but spoiler alert, they're ALREADY suffering, and they want to help. So LET THEM.

Find your person (or people).

This is not a path you should walk alone. Have your person ready to go to doctor's appointments, to talk when you need them, to be your Support Team of One. For me, this was my husband, PJ, who is just the best damn human on earth. He took off work. He canceled fishing trips. He postponed plans. He went with me to *every* fucking appointment, and I am so grateful for that.

Initially, I was like, "Oh, you don't need to do that. I'll be fine." Because, you know, I'm independent and self-reliant, and I wasn't about to admit I didn't have something managed, even when I didn't.

Because I wasn't fine.

Going to the doctor to talk about cancer, your own mortality, and all the suckiest treatment plans is absolutely terrible. It's terrifying. It's horrifying.

This was not the time in my life to be plucky and independent.

I needed someone there. I was never in a million years going to ask for someone to be there, but PJ volunteered. I told him he didn't have to because, like many women walking this earth, I felt like the best thing I could do was make myself small and convenient, to absolutely never be a bother to anyone.

He insisted. I'm so glad he did.

PJ canceled business trips. He even canceled a going to a BBQ competition in Kansas City (he's on a competitive team that's been together for years), and he canceled lunches with friends. He was with me at every appointment, holding my hand.

I thought I wouldn't need it.

But, God, did I need it.

So, this is not a time to be demure and mindful, okay? Save that bullshit for your social media page. Right now, get Your Person, or Your People, on rotation and take someone with you even if you think you don't need it.

Especially if you think you don't need it.

If you're like me, accepting help, or admitting I even need it in the first place, feels almost more terrifying than cancer. I've prided myself on being self-sufficient my whole life. I've always been independent, fiercely so, and was a single mom of two for nine years. Asking for help felt like failure.

But it's not.

I know you think you've got this, and you do, but have a trusted person go with you. Your spouse. Your best friend. Your cousin. YOUR PERSON.

You would not—unless you're a masochist—go to a haunted house alone, and you shouldn't go to your oncologist's office alone either. It's got more jump scares than any abandoned amusement park. I swear to God, I'd prefer killer clowns jumping out of a dark corner than being told they aren't sure if I need a lumpectomy or a mastectomy, or radiation, or also chemo.

Do not go through this alone. I know you may not have a choice, but if it's at all possible, don't go alone.

I'll give you several good reasons:

1. There aren't extra prizes or accolades for "not being a bother" when it comes to your fucking cancer appointments. This is a time when you SHOULD be a fucking bother. You've got fucking CANCER. If you can't call in your chips now, WHEN can you? What are you saving them for? You want to die with a whole lot of "I never asked anyone for anything like a fool" trading cards? You can't lean on your people or call in favors when you're dead.

2. Letting people help isn't selfish. It can be *good* for them, actually. There's something called the Helper's High.[18] That's when you feel good when you help someone else in need. We've come down too hard on people lately for virtue signaling by posting every nice thing they've ever done online, but the science proves that when you actually do something selfless and thoughtful for someone, you feel good about yourself. Being supportive and nice actually releases warm and fuzzy hormones in our brains. Spoiler: that's because you did a good deed. And good deeds are good—for the people we help and for us.

3. If you're like me, sometimes, when I hear bad news, I simply tune out. Remember that white room I talked about? My self-defense mechanism when someone tells me I need to have my boob chopped off is simply to

---

[18] "The Helper's High" by Larry Dossey, *Explore*, Volume 14, Issue 6, November 2018.

opt not to hear it. So, I needed another set of ears in there, so I could ask, "What the hell just happened?" Or, that person—like my amazing husband PJ—will crack a joke at just the right time, so I laugh instead of faint. He's amazing at that.

4. Sometimes, all you want is a fucking witness, someone living the horror with you, so you can commiserate. Your person may ALSO be scared to death in that room and may, actually, not get all the information either. PJ turned to me after one doctor's visit and said, "What the hell just happened?" And then we laughed. BOTH of us went into the white room, and that's okay, too. Because I had someone there, with me, on that gut-wrenching plunge on the roller coaster, and we could both laugh about how scary the fucking ride really was. Sometimes, you just want a witness with you, someone to confirm that, yes, this shit is fucking terrifying.

So, your person might be your spouse, or it might be your sister or brother, or best friend. It doesn't matter who it is. It doesn't even matter if you have a rotating team of Your People. Take someone to every appointment. To be there, to hold your hand or crack a joke, or to take notes when the doctor or nurse is talking, so you can safely escape into your white room.

You, of course, get to decide whether Your Person is in the exam room, or in the waiting room, or in the damn parking lot. Just bring Your Person.

Delegate. Seriously. For real this time.

You're going to need to get some shit off your plate. This whole Superwoman/Wonder Woman/Captain Marvel shit you've been doing your whole life of balancing your career/ family responsibilities/friends' regular brunch/book club/not letting the house devolve into the worst episode of *Hoarders* all while NOT sleeping a wink WILL NOT FLY.

Time for you to delegate the shit that you can.

Cleaning? Let the kids do it. Even if they do it poorly. They load the dishwasher horribly and only half of them come out clean? Who cares. Let it go.

Could this meeting really be an email? Then, do it.

Do you really need to go to that condo board or home-owners association meeting? Maybe you could skip this one. Can the PTA do the bake sale this year without you? They *can* grab a tray of donuts from the grocery bakery and be done with it.

You are going to need every ounce of strength to FIGHT FOR YOUR LIFE, and you do not have time to get waylaid by silly bullshit that doesn't matter. And here's a hint: most of it is silly bullshit.

Back when you were healthy and not facing your own mortality, you could volunteer to do boring shit at the school, stay late at work to help out your helpless coworker, or pick up the slack when your spouse forgot a kid's birthday.

Not now.

Everyone has to pull their own weight now.

You've been floating some people. I know you have.

Well, it's time for a Come to Jesus meeting because Fighting Cancer has jumped to the top of your to-do list and that messy bitch is not going anywhere. Time for some kids to figure out how to do their own laundry. Or your spouse to cook a few more meals. Or maybe you buy paper plates and never wash another plate again until your treatment is over.

However you can delegate, do it.

Delegating is good for you AND them.

And you know what? It's better for EVERYONE. If you've been carrying some people (like your grown son who still has never cooked a meal in his life), well, he'll finally learn to make mac and cheese, and that will be a good thing.

You're not failing as a mother; you are succeeding in giving your kids (no matter what their ages) some more responsibilities.

Your spouse who relies on you to go to the grocery store and doesn't know how the self-checkout works? Well, they are going to learn and it's going to be amazing.

That clueless boss who leans on you to look good? She'll finally have to stand on her own two feet in meetings. It'll be fantastic.

Also, bonus—the people in your life who love you want to do things. They might be terrible at doing these things and they might mix white and red clothes in the washer, but then they'll learn.

Don't pretend that you can still do everything you could do before you got the diagnosis. You can't. And that's okay.
I wanted desperately to hang on to the illusion that cancer was not going to slow me down. I had a book to finish and a new book to promote. Cancer, gosh darn it, wasn't going to get in the way.

Oh, it got in the way. Big fucking time.

I'm not sure how I thought a needle to the armpit *wouldn't* get all the attention and that waiting for biopsy results *might* make it difficult to concentrate on writing *fucking romantic comedies*, but, I mean, I'm a diehard optimist.

We've established cancer is a messy bitch, and she does splash into her life screaming, "Me! Me! Me! It's all about ME!" This means you will need help doing things. Especially after treatment starts. Some days you'll feel like you're walking through twelve inches of mud in the rain.

You're going to need people to help you. They're not going to do things exactly the way you want. And that's okay.

You might have a particular way you like to do things. Well, they might not get done that way. The towels might not be folded just so. The sheets? Not changed as often on the bed. Dinner might not be what you wanted to make. Someone might leave a streak of Windex on the mirror when they clean. They might put the toilet paper roll on backward.

But you know what?

So what.

You've got bigger fish to fry. You've got bigger problems right now. You need your rest, and people are going to offer their (maybe not perfect) help but take it.

Ask for you what you need.

This one is a hard one. So many of us women have been trained our whole lives to turn away help. "Oh, no, I'm fine, thank you" or "I've got this, but thank you!" or "Really, that's not necessary!"

I've met some cancer patients who believe their very lives—the stress and unfairness in it—gave them cancer.

I'm not sure about that, but some studies show that stress can help grow your cancer faster because cancer—literally—eats that stuff up.[19]

So unless you want to give your cancer an all-you-can-eat buffet, now is the time NOT to stress about stupid shit that never merited the stress to begin with. Of course, don't stress about being stressed, okay?

Now is just the time you're going to need help, and you SHOULD ask for it.

Be specific.

---

[19] Markham Heid, "How Stress Affects Cancer Risk," MD Anderson Cancer Center, December 2014.

Assign tasks to friends, neighbors, and relatives.

Can your best friend pick up your kids from school? Check.

Can your mother-in-law get some of her friends together to handle meals for a couple of nights a week?

Can you ask a coworker to help pick up some of your slack? Can you get your boss on board with delegating some of your workload?

Can your spouse take over dishes for a little while?

Can your teenage daughter walk the dog?

These things might seem small. One task here. Another there. But if you ask people to help—and many people will WANT to help—and assign them tasks, you can get things off your plate, STRESS LESS, and focus on resting, getting healthier, and the fight ahead.

If you're like me, you never ask anyone for anything and would rather jump out of an airplane with a wonky parachute than admit you don't have everything under control.

Well, this is the one time you don't have everything under control.

Because. . . I cannot say this enough. . . it's fucking CAN-CER. Nobody has a handle on CANCER.

At least, not at first.

Not yet.

And that's okay.

Because as soon as you whip cancer's ass, you will be back to being a control-freak who turns down every offer of help and stresses about what to make for dinner.

You're going to need every single bit of that stubborn, my-way-is-the-best-way, don't-fold-towels-like-that, scrub-the-dishes-before-you-put-them-in-the-dishwasher energy to beat cancer. Let other people handle the small things you fret about. Set your control-freakish focus, that single-minded nagging, on your cancer. Nag that shit to death. Tell that malignant son of

77

a bitch just all the ways it got it wrong, and shame it into leaving your body forever.

When friends/relatives/neighbors/coworkers volunteer help you DON'T want, it's okay to say that.

The only thing worse than asking for help is feeling like you can't turn down help that will absolutely make things worse but that someone else is generously offering.

Look, people in your life are going to want to help, and maybe sometimes they have terrible ideas.

Maybe your mother-in-law says she'll move in with you and watch the kids, except that your mother-in-law always criticizes you 24-7 and the thought of her under your roof makes you want the cancer to kill you faster.

Some people need permission to turn others down, so consider this your official permission: you don't have to accept help if it's going to make things worse.

The whole point of help is to make things better.

If your coworker who burns everything she touches and makes meals that taste like hot garbage offers you dinner five nights a week, you can steer her to a DoorDash gift card instead.

If your father-in-law volunteers to come clean out the gutters, but he's way too wobbly on a ladder and the last thing you need is an elderly man with a broken hip on your lawn, you can tell him, "Actually, could you drive the kids to school instead?"

If the busybody of the neighborhood wants to go with you to every doctor's appointment so she can get the scoop and share it with every single person she meets, you can say no.

You can always say no.

Say no, early and often, if the help being offered isn't going to actually help.

There's a fine line here because some of the help offered you might think you don't need, but you actually desperately do.

My friends put together a calendar where each of them brought me a meal during my week of surgery. Initially, I didn't think we'd need this—my husband cooks (amazingly) and my teen daughters also tinker in the kitchen. But it turned out the meals were a lifesaver because I was recovering, and both my husband and kids were exhausted too (from the stress of my surgery, from picking up slack around the house, and just generally living with the messy bitch that is breast cancer because she is a A LOT).

If I'd said no to the meal train too early, then I wouldn't have gained the benefit of having the meals when I needed them.

Also, mealtime was especially stressful in my house because we're a blended family of seven, and we've got several omnivores, one picky carnivore, and two pescatarians. It was almost impossible to make anything that everyone could all agree on, or get excited about, but during that week when I wasn't making the meals, well, they couldn't really complain. It wasn't *my* doing. It was my friends, they were being nice, and I was sick. And. . . well, just having them NOT complain was a gift in and of itself.

Sucking it up and eating a delicious new shrimp and tomato dish was something they'd have to try or suddenly THEY were the problem.

So—accept the help that eases your stress and decline the help that increases it.

It's okay—at any time—to ask people to step up—or step down.

This road ahead is bumpy, and the treatment—whatever you decide—will be challenging. It's okay to ask friends or relatives to step up—or step down—if you need help OR if you need different help than what you're getting.

If in the middle of that meal train, it becomes too stressful and not helpful, ask your friends to hit pause.

If your sister watching your kids after school has become a nightmare because she loads them up with sugar and junk food, you can ask her NOT to do that, or you can ask her to pause.

Just because someone is helping you out of the goodness of their heart, it doesn't mean you can't request things. Or change things. Or hit the pause button. The whole point is getting the help you need and not the help you don't.

Pep talk #5:

Hey, Warrior. How you doing? Just checking in on you and making sure you're not trying to do this all alone and not be a bother to anyone.

You're worth being a bother. You're worth getting the help. You DESERVE the help. How many times have you helped others? How often have you come to the aid of friends or family? You've put yourself out there to help neighbors and coworkers more times than you can count.

Now it's time for them to help you.

You'd do the same for them. And you probably already have. Accept the help with gratitude and grace because you're freaking amazing and people want to help you.

Accepting the help doesn't mean you've failed or you're lesser than. It means you're an outstanding human with fantastic family and friends.

Who wouldn't want to help you?

Chapter Six

Manage Your Stress Before It Manages You

"The mind is everything. What you think you become."

—Buddha

"Let's take that again," said the nurse at the infusion center, where I'm scheduled to get my weekly round of chemotherapy, as she unwraps the blood pressure cuff from my arm and sends me a worried glance. My blood pressure just spiked high enough to warrant a trip to urgent care, and she's concerned. "Normally, I'd think about sending you to the ER for this reading."

Even my husband, PJ, who takes medicine for his chronically high blood pressure, said, "What was that reading again?" He frowns at the numbers. "That's way too high, babe."

"This happens anytime I come here," I joke, and it's true. Now, several months into cancer treatment, my heart rate skyrockets anytime I see a white coat.

"You know medical anxiety is a real thing," the nurse tells me. "It happens to people."

It's definitely happening to me.

Every single time I go in for a chemo treatment, I have a high blood pressure reading. I'm voluntarily getting poison pumped in my veins, so I guess my body is just acting accordingly.

This shit is not for the faint of heart.

And the thing is—I bet before diagnosis, your life wasn't a stress-free cakewalk. I bet you were ALREADY stressed with all the things women are always stressed about: work, family, finances, friends, spouses, aging parents, aging friends, never-enough retirement funds, and what the hell to cook for dinner (my least favorite decision of the day). You are probably already well acquainted with stress, with insomnia, with anxiety.

And now. . . fucking cancer? Are you shitting me, universe? And even worse, stress makes the cancer grow faster? Hello? How can I NOT be stressed? I have fucking cancer.

I hate to be the one to break it to you, but the stress and worry crushing you this whole time is about to get a hundred times worse. And the stress will be here to stay for weeks and months, maybe even years. It's good for the cancer and bad for you; it even increases your risk of dying from cancer.[20] So, you're going to have to find a way to manage it, before it manages you.

People handle stress differently. I hit the treadmill and watched horror movies. (I might have breast cancer, but at least I didn't have a psychopath chasing me with a chainsaw. Point, me.) Also, there was something amazingly refreshing about watching the Last Girl in the horror movie escape. How did she do it? How did *she* overcome her fear? Watching Girl-Escapes-Psychotic-Killer movies was a blueprint for how I planned to face my own fear.

Also, my counselor felt like I was trying to escape my life, and maybe I was. I'm sure there's some clear psychological analysis to be done here.

But the good news is you don't have to watch horror movies to relieve stress. There are things that work. Here are some (less scary) things that helped me.

---

[20] Matthew Solan, "Prolonged stress may increase the risk of death from cancer," *Harvard Health Publishing*, Harvard Medical School, January 1, 2023.

Meditate

Don't knock it until you've tried it. Download one of those apps like Headspace, or whichever one you prefer, and try a few minutes of meditation. This is one way to get a handle on a lot of things, but it's also a pathway to just sit in the moment, not rush ahead to the future or the past. In the present moment, you are alive. You are not dead. You are not in surgery. You are not getting radiation or chemo. Sitting in your bedroom, your study, or your kitchen, you are simply alive in this moment, and the terrible treatment scaring you to death isn't actually happening yet.

Being in the moment might seem like somewhere you DON'T want to be when you have breast cancer. It's counterintuitive. But your fear is what's COMING next, not what is NOW. I always went down a deep rabbit hole of what-if: What if the surgery went badly? What if they found more cancer? What if chemo was a living hell? The what-ifs are a lot scarier than the now. In the now, I felt fine. No one sat in my living room, poking me with a needle. I wasn't getting chemo or anything else. The cancer itself didn't hurt. It was all the treatments that threatened to torture me.

Short-circuit that fear by breathing, being in the moment, being in your body, being alive, and not being in the middle of all those horrible things on the horizon.

But I tried meditating that one time, you say, and I sucked at it!

Here's a hint: Everyone sucks at meditating. Everyone gets distracted. Everybody fails to hit the sweet spot of perfect, thought-free, calm existence in the moment.

Being *good* at meditating isn't what meditating is all about.

Meditating is about *slowing down* your brain. It's about trying not to worry about a million other things and just sit in the moment. Your brain is always getting ahead of itself—thinking about the next treatment, tomorrow, next year, whether you're going to have enough money for retirement, whether you'll need to get a second job. Worry, worry, worry. . . about *the future.*

Meditating makes the brain focus on *right now*, and right now will likely be boring compared to all the imagined horrors your brain might be cooking up in your future.

You don't have to be good at meditating for it to work and to get the benefits of it. You just need the patience to keep trying. Just the act of trying to wrangle your brain away from future fears and worries gives you benefits.

I also happen to have an amazing friend who does guided meditations. She also does aura readings (don't hate it until you've tried it). She was kind enough to do guided meditations with me that helped me get to the core of some of the emotional weight I was carrying.

Freeing. Amazing. Fantastic.

She and my counselor helped me get my mind in the right place before major surgery.

Don't forget to breathe.

Breathing might sound like a dumb way to treat stress, but let me tell you something: when you're sitting in that damn windowless room getting the worst news of your life, there will be plenty of times you'll forget to breathe at all.

There's a very specific kind of breathing—triangle breathing—that helps reduce stress and fool your brain and body into lowering stress hormones. Triangle breathing is simple:

Breathe in for three seconds.

Hold for three seconds.

Breathe out for three seconds.

This shit does actually work. Because when you're stressed and in fight-or-flight mode, you typically breath shallowly or not at all, readying your body for action. Long breaths tell your nervous system to stand down. Slow breathing calms your system down and says there's no saber-tooth about to leap, that you don't have to run for your life.[21]

Make your own epic playlist.

Look, I love music. I love all kinds of genres of music. I believe in the power of music.

And right now, if you're going to stay sane, you're going to need the epic playlist of your life.

Pile on fight songs (you'll need the courage), throw on some sad ones too (because this shit IS sad and tragic), and definitely get some angry ones on there (because WTF?!). I'm not going to tell you what music to listen to, and you may have very different tastes than mine, but I encourage all the songs that curse ("NSFW" by Psychostick is 100% cursing). Break-up songs work particularly well for your playlist because you have been betrayed—by your own body. And you are breaking up with cancer. ("Irreplaceable" by Beyoncé and "Fighter" by Christina Aguilera).

Find songs that get you pumped. (Yacht rock? Why the fuck not?)

So, it all works.

Pick your own favorite songs. Find the ones that speak to you that get you pumped. You're going to need to psyche yourself up, my friend. You're going to need to get yourself ready for the fight of your life, and music is the best, fastest way to do that.

Get your playlist.

Add to it.

---

[21] Andrea Zaccaro, Andrea Piarulli, Marco Laurino, Erika Garbella, Danilo Menicucci, Bruno Neri, Angelo Gemignani, "How Breath-Control Can Change Your Life: A Systematic Review on Psycho-Physiological Correlates of Slow Breathing," *Frontiers in Human Neuroscience*, September 7, 2018.

Change it.

Listen to it.

I know the last thing you thought someone would recommend post-cancer diagnosis is for you to make yourself a mixtape. But here we are.

On this journey, this road I never planned to be on, music helped me in profound ways. When I didn't think I was strong enough, I found strength in music. When I was sad, I was able to cry to music, and when I was angry, I was able to shout to music.

I love music. I believe it taps directly into our emotional selves (which happen to be a total wreck right now). I made multiple playlists, but the first one I called "Fuck Cancer," and I put two kinds of songs on it: fight songs and fuck-off songs. This was my amped-up, fuck-everyone, I-won't-back-down list. I needed this list when I needed to get amped up, like Rocky before a fight, when I was hitting a low and needed to get pumped up. You'll be amazed how many break-up songs work just fine for sending cancer a middle finger. They get right to the heart of the betrayal you're feeling. It's not your significant other who betrayed you, it's your own body, and that somehow makes the betrayal worse.

Also, science tells us that music helps alleviate stress.[22] But I bet you know this already.

So fill up that list with all your favorite songs, whatever they may be, about betrayal and recovery from a broken heart. Who cares if your spouse or kids think the music or artist is dumb? This is the music in *your* earbuds, okay?

Fill that playlist with all the angry songs because you are fucking angry. Furious. At cancer. At your body. At everyone and everything.

---

[22] Donald Collins, "The Power of Music to Reduce Stress," PsychCentral, August 18, 2021.

Blast this playlist while you hit the treadmill, go for a walk, or do the dishes. Move around while you listen to it, get that anger out. Punch a punching bag. Scrub a pot until it gleams. Peloton the shit out of that bike.

You can't stay angry forever, but you'll need somewhere to put that anger. You'll need to get it out, and music helps with that. If you've got train tracks near your house, go stand under them and scream. You're mad as hell. You should be mad as hell.

Cancer is a fucking asshole. An asshole that completely upended your life.

Fuck cancer.

Be mad at it.

You earned the right.

If an actual person came to your doorstep, rang the doorbell, and told you that he planned to take thousands of dollars from you, make you worry you'd lose your life, scare all your family members, then you'd want to put that man in jail for life.

That's what cancer does.

So get that angry playlist going.

And then, also, get that sad playlist going.

The one packed with all the songs that make you want to cry. The sad ones. Because you'll also need that playlist, too. The sad, woe-is-me playlist. I called mine the "Time to Cry" playlist, and I played it on a speaker while I showered, took a bath, or was in the car when no one was around. I cried a lot.

This doesn't mean you're weak, by the way.

Crying does amazing and wonderful things in your body. It releases oxytocin and endorphins to help ease physical and emotional pain and help you feel better (I bet you all already know this), but according to researchers at Yale University, crying also helps restore emotional balance (and in the middle of a cancer battle, we need all the balance we can get).[23,24]

You probably will too, and sometimes, you just need songs that help you do that. That give you permission to do that.

Music is wonderful. Get your playlist together. Add to it. Find new artists and new songs that can help you through this time.

Music shows us we're not alone in our pain or sadness or anger. Others are right there with us.

Get Healthy

I know this sounds ridiculous.

You want me to get in shape? I've got CANCER.

I get it.

Let me explain.

The first oncologist I saw his first question to me was: "How's your health?"

"Okay, I guess, aside from the *cancer*," I responded. I mean what was I supposed to say? I had cancer. How was my health? Bitch, please.

In an instant, that diagnosis takes you from "healthy" to "sick." Even though you probably don't feel sick.

You feel fine.

It's all the treatments that will make you feel like shit.

But more on that later.

Back to getting in shape and your health. That not-so-great-with-the-bedside-manner oncologist was *trying* to tell me

---

[23] Ashley Marcin, "9 Ways Crying May Benefit Your Health," Healthline, April 15, 2017.
[24] Oriana R Aragón, Margaret S Clark, Rebecca L Dyer, John A Bargh, "Dimorphous expressions of positive emotion: displays of both care and aggression in response to cute stimuli," *Psychological Science Journal*, January 27, 2015.

that my outcomes—whichever treatment plan in store for me—would be better the healthier I was going into them.

This is just medical fact.

The healthier you are going into surgery, chemo, radiation, or anything else, the less likely you'll have complications.

So, I know it feels like an oxymoron: *I've been diagnosed with cancer, and so I need to exercise, eat right, quit smoking, and cut back on drinking? What the fuck? I've got cancer. How can I even be healthy? Are you serious right now?*

Um, yeah. I am.

I know you don't want to.

When I got my cancer diagnosis, I wallowed in pity, ate shitty food, drank too much, and wanted to give a middle finger to my body. And did. Often. She'd betrayed me. She'd let me down, so why would I become one of those people who ate just two bites of quinoa and kale, bragging about triathlons? The last thing I wanted to do was get in shape, even though, honestly, I'd let myself go.

I used to head to the gym. I used to try to kind of eat right (with several cheat days of course). But then the COVID pandemic upended everything. The world went into lockdown, so no more gym. No more run/walking the occasional 5K. Quarantine passed, and I could've gotten back into the gym and eating right, but I just didn't. I felt like, well, I tried. I turned fifty and I started to convince myself that the extra twenty pounds I was carrying was just the natural aging process.

After all, when do we get to let ourselves go? Was I supposed to be running 5Ks and worrying about carbs when I'm seventy? Eighty? Ninety? At some point, can I just take my foot off the gas and relax?

My grandmother, who died of COVID at age ninety-seven, still worried about dieting well into her nineties. I vowed I wasn't going to be like that. At some point, I was just going to eat what I want, sit on my ass, and stream shit. Body image be damned.

And then, cancer fucked that plan all up.

Because I knew I was out of shape. I was the most out of shape I'd been my whole life, and now, I had cancer. Did I blame myself? Maybe. But, I also knew that I was looking at treatment that was going to be physically hard. Surgery. Chemo, maybe. Radiation, maybe. And going into that out of shape probably wasn't the smartest idea.

So how *was* my health?

Piss poor. I ate too many carbs. I drank too much. I binged on pizza and take-out. My only exercise was walking the dog at his very slow, sniff-everything pace.

Plus, I was stressed the fuck out. I was a hurricane of emotions, most of which were black-out fear.

As animals, when we're afraid, our bodies pump all those fight or flight chemicals like cortisol into our veins that allow our body to move quickly in emergency situations.[25] Our ancestors used cortisol to fight the saber-tooth or flee to safety, but how do you fight or flight a visit to the oncologist's office? You don't. You have to sit there, not throwing punches or running away, and listen to someone in a white lab coat tell you that every treatment option for you is shitty, painful, and tortuous. You don't leap into action (thereby dissolving the harmful hormones and chemicals). Instead, you just sit with them, and they in turn contribute to high blood pressure, clogged arteries, and a host of other unhealthy things.

I didn't feel great sitting with these stress chemicals, so I hit the treadmill.

---

[25] Howard E. LeWine, MD, "Understanding the stress response, Chronic activation of this survival mechanism impairs health," *Harvard Health Publishing*, April 3, 2024.

I'd gotten the treadmill with the best of intentions during COVID, but it had become the most expensive laundry rack ever.

I used to run 5Ks before the pandemic, and I was determined to run them again. Oh, hitting that treadmill hurt. It hurt bad. But, I kind of felt like, that's right, body. I'm punishing you.

You mess with me? I'm gonna mess with you.

I blasted my angry rock, my betrayal breakup songs, and pounded that treadmill. Each angry step I took was a fuck you to cancer. To the universe. To all the things that brought me here.

I'd be pouring sweat. Angry.

I'd cry.

I'd shout.

I'd pound that treadmill.

Repeat.

There was nowhere else to put my anger, so I shed it through sweat and tears.

And afterward, I felt... not good. But better. Less likely that I was going to curl up in the fetal position in the corner and cry. I got all those endorphins from exercising. And, I got the bonus feeling of beating up my body because I was so damn mad at it.

It might not have been the best mental health option, but it was better than knocking up the local liquor store or shouting at people in traffic.

So, I recommend it.

I ran. I lifted weights. I did core work because I *fucking hate* core work, and it was the best way I could think of to punish my body.

But also? You know what? When I got a double mastectomy, I was SO grateful for all that core work. Because I used my stomach to get myself in and out of bed, not my arms or chest, where it was all hurt and swollen.

All those times I had sore muscles, and I thought *Good, body, you deserve that pain.* Well, you know what? When I had real pain from surgery, I was USED to beating up my body. I was. . . kind of. . . oddly. . . ready for pain. I think my pain tolerance was higher because I'd had all those sore muscles leading up to surgery.

And then it hit me: I wasn't actually punishing my body at all. I was *preparing* it. I was working it hard so that I could bounce back faster.

So, move your body. It doesn't have to be on a treadmill. It can be a walk around the block. It can be stomach crunches in your den.

Blast your angry tunes. Or your sad ones.

Shout. Cry.

Get it out.

Don't let it fester inside you. Be mad at your body. Work it, hard.

Eat right. Punish it with salads and leafy greens and lean protein.

Because I'll tell you, after eight weeks of working out and eating right, an amazing thing happened. I got back to running five kilometers before I had my surgery. My lungs were good. My heart was great. I was ready for surgery. Like, healthy and ready.

And, I *felt* ready. I felt like I'd done all I could do to get my body ready for the trauma of surgery, and so I felt calm the night before my double mastectomy. I didn't worry about my heart giving out on the operating table. I didn't worry about not waking up from anesthesia.

In the eight weeks from diagnosis to surgery, I'd gotten in shape, as good a shape as I could manage, and I felt calm going into surgery. An amazing thing happened: I had a complication-free recovery. No infections, no setbacks. Quick healing. My body came through it like a fucking champ.

My counselor told me that my body showed up for me because I showed up for it.

All this time, I thought I was punishing my body, but in reality, I was raining tough love down on it to get it ready for the hard road ahead. All the time I thought I was hating on my body I actually was loving on it.

My surgery, including two mastectomies and partial reconstruction, took five hours. I was intubated and spent at least a week after that trying to get my lung capacity back to normal. I don't want to even think about how that recovery would've been if I hadn't gotten into shape.

I didn't let my body waste away on the couch, eating pints of ice cream, though I badly wanted to.

I got it in shape, to give it the best chance at the best outcome.

I showed up for my body, and it showed up for me.

And that's how this works.

Remember: cancer doesn't get to decide. It doesn't get to decide you're weak or out of shape or unhealthy.

You can be healthy. Even with cancer. Fuck cancer.

So move your body. Get in shape. Get it ready for what lies ahead because the road is full of potholes and fire, and you've got Mt. Everest in front of you.

One caveat: don't run a marathon straight out of the gate if this is your first time exercising in your life. Start slowly—start with walks. Don't overdo it. Work your body at a pace that makes logical sense, or you'll end up throwing your back out.

The most important thing is to show up for your body.

So it will show up for you.

Talk to Someone Who's Paid to Listen

Your body isn't going to be able to fight unless your mind is right.

I began counseling shortly after I was diagnosed. I went back to the counselor who helped me during another acute time in my life—when I got divorced. It felt like serendipity because she'd moved away to Florida, and she'd just moved back to Illinois a month before I was diagnosed.

I don't know how you all feel about counseling, but I found it SO important during this process. A counselor shouldn't tell you what to do, or which treatments are best for you, but they should help you get to a decision—even a hard decision—that you feel strongly about. That's what my counselor did for me.

I know a lot of people have a lot of feelings about support groups and therapists, but I'll tell you what my therapist told me: "Weak people don't come to see me. The strong ones do."

She helped me reframe some of the problems I was facing: Was I letting fear drive? Or was I rationally making healthcare decisions? She helped me unpack some of my issues (why didn't I want to accept help from others?). She helped me focus my frustration and fear, telling me that nobody expected me to be a damn gazelle. I had every right to be a bull in a china shop as long as I kept on moving and made it to the other side.

I highly recommend going to see someone. There's a LOT of emotional baggage that comes along with a cancer diagnosis, and it's important to feel and unpack it all. If you don't, if you skip this step, you'll be less clear-eyed about your own healthcare decisions, and there's a good chance when the treatment is all over, and you're given the all-clear, you suddenly find yourself mired in a deep, hole of depression.

The feelings will catch up to you, no matter how hard you run from them. Might as well get them all out now, deal with them as they come up so that they don't landslide into your life later. One in four cancer patients experience depression, and this can come at any time–with diagnosis, or even after treatment is over.[26]

I don't know how you feel about counseling and therapy. Maybe you hate it. Maybe you love it.

But, I'm going to tell you right now: your greatest weapon in this fight for your life is your mind. I think counseling is the best option for this, but it could also be your best girlfriend, your spouse, or a support group, whomever can help you reframe a problem, be your support, but also give you a kick in the butt when you need it.

Throughout this whole process, there were plenty of times I wanted to pout and DID pout. I wanted to sit down and scream, "I don't wanna!" just like I was two again, throwing a tantrum. I needed my counselor to help me see that's exactly what I was doing.

It's okay to pout. It's okay not to want to go to the doctor or get the treatment or face the reality. But eventually, we have to. Sometimes, we'll have to drag ourselves kicking and screaming through this whole damn process.

You've got to get your head right. Because cancer loves to live in your head. It loves to fuck with you. Keep you up at night. Rile up your anxiety. Make you second-guess everything.

As I mentioned before, I had an amazing counselor who popped back into my life exactly when I needed her most. I point this out because there are going to be times in this journey where you might feel like the universe, God, or whatever, is out to get you. That you are being punished, that everything is horrible, and it's all darkness with no light.

But, the universe, or whatever you believe in, also gives you little breaks. Little uplifting moments that you might not expect. It puts people in your path that will help you so much

---

[26] "Depression," American Cancer Society, July 24, 2025.

(the very first infusion nurse I had for chemo was literally sent by an angel).

Yes, you're going through a horrible time, and cancer fucking sucks.

But it's also true that you might find little bits of light, bursts of joy, wrapped up in perfect packages just for you. Just keep on the lookout for them because they'll be a lifeline. More on this later.

My counselor—moving back to the area after being gone for years—was one such gift from the universe. My counselor had personal experience with cancer. She'd had cervical cancer, and she'd also counseled so many women who were going through breast cancer. She had the expertise and the knowledge.

She's the one who first told me cancer doesn't get to decide. That very piece of advice was a lifeline. She's the one who pointed out that I could be a victim. Or I could be a survivor. That it was my mindset that could determine how well I come out of this. Or, hell, *if* I come out of this.

She helped me reframe, and understand, the problem I was facing, so that I could really get the best treatment for me.

Cancer seems so big, so insurmountable, and it knocks even the strongest of us on our asses. But it's not the end-all, be-all. It's not all powerful. We can take our power back, and part of that is getting your head right.

Get Spiritual

I don't know about the god you pray to, or if you pray at all, but this can be a time for many to get spiritual, or lean on their faith. I'm not going to tell you how to do this. You probably already know what works best for you.

In difficult times, it helps to connect to the universe on a deeper, more spiritual level, so that we can draw on the strength we need.

Attitude Actually Is Everything

I know a lot of people have told you about how important a positive attitude is, and this may make you want to puke. I get it.

Before I had my double-mastectomy, the doctor flat out told me that there are mountains of studies that say a patient who believes they will be fine will turn out to be fine, and those that don't, typically aren't fine at all.

But, let's dig deeper into "positive attitude" because I don't think this means you have to walk around like everything is wonderful and this is the best time of your life.

Hell, no. You've got fucking *cancer*.

Nobody skips through having cancer, smiling, laughing, and having no trouble with it. I'm not talking about being Mary Poppins. I'm talking about being Uma Thurman in *Kill Bill*.

A positive attitude can take a lot of forms. Personally, some days, my positive attitude was two middle fingers to cancer.

My positive attitude was angry. It was, "Who the hell does cancer think she is? She's not getting away with this, and she's going to wish she never met me."

That's a positive attitude.

Sometimes, my positive attitude was simply admitting I was scared shitless. Admitting you're scared helps you deal with it.

You don't have to get through this like a graceful gazelle. You can snap at people. You can be irritable. You can be depressed. You can be scared.

You just have to keep moving.

Having a positive attitude doesn't mean being delusional, thinking everything is sunshine and roses. Having a positive attitude means believing in *you*. It means feeling, deep down in your bones, that you ARE going to kick this.

You're going to do it for your spouse.

Your family.

Your friends.

But most of all—most importantly of all—you're going to do it FOR YOURSELF.

Pep talk #6:

Hey, Soldier. Feeling stressed out? Totally get it. Been there. Take care of yourself in all the ways you can.

Remember that worry is like a rocking chair. It gives you something to do but it doesn't get you anywhere. Figure out the ways to reduce your stress so you can have the best attitude possible in these impossible times.

Upside to all this? Once you manage the impossible stress of cancer, you'll be like a superhero in your remission life. Things that stressed you out before (Bills? Kids? Aging Parents?)? Please. You've faced worse. Those things will seem small. Once you manage the stress of cancer, you can manage almost anything.

Stress distracts you from the real fight.

Tackle stress with the same relentlessness you tackle cancer.

Chapter Seven

Not All Doctors Are Good. Get A Team of Avengers, Not the Three Stooges

"You define your own life. Don't let other people or your circumstances write your script."

—Oprah Winfrey

My dad, the retired orthopedic surgeon, has a favorite joke:

You know what they call the person who graduates last in their med school class?

Doctor.

Not all doctors are the same. Not all hospitals are the same. We do not, actually, have the best healthcare system in the world, despite what the American propaganda machine has been telling you—especially if you live far from a city or in a poor neighborhood.

I don't mention this to add to your anxiety.

I mention this so that you're fully armed with all the knowledge, so you can advocate for yourself. So you don't just nod at whatever your provider tells you. That you become your own best cheerleader for the best care.

According to a recent Commonwealth Fund study, our healthcare system—regardless of where you live—is one of the most expensive in the world, and yet we're sicker than people in other industrialized nations, we die younger, and we have a harder time affording even basic healthcare.[27]

In the Commonwealth Fund study, the United States ranked last on access to care and health outcomes (including acute illnesses, chronic disease, and DEATH) compared to other nations like Germany, Canada, France, Australia, the UK, and the Netherlands. When we put ourselves beside them, we Americans live the shortest lives and face the most avoidable deaths. There are a myriad of reasons for these stats, but they're facts.

Also, a third of Americans reported receiving an error in treatment, a wrong medication or dose of medication, an incorrect result for a test, or had delays in getting test results. This is among the highest rate of mistakes in the world.[28]

So, unlike other countries where you can put your care on autopilot and trust you'll be taken care of, in America you need to be a strong advocate for yourself and you need to pay attention. You can't just trust that the system will work fine for you because it might not.

If you're a person of color, then you have to advocate EVEN harder for yourself because the bias in medicine is real, and, no joke, the bias can cost you your life. No matter what you've been trained to think, there's a real disparity in care.[29] So, this is the time to raise your hand, ask questions, and pester your healthcare team.

---

[27] David Blumenthal, Evan D. Gumas, Arnav Shah, Munira Z. Gunja, Reginald D. Williams II, "Mirror, Mirror 2024: A Portrait of the Failing U.S. Health System," The Commonwealth Fund, September 19, 2024.

[28] "International Survey: U.S. Leads in Medical Errors," The Commonwealth Fund, Nov 03, 2005.

[29] Juanita J Chinn, Iman K Martin, Nicole Redmond, "Health Equity Among Black Women in the United States," *Journal of Women's Health*, February 2021.

The good news is, because breast cancer is so damn common, there typically are systems in place to treat it. Your insurance company hopefully shouldn't deny reconstruction surgery (which is enshrined in federal and most state laws), and your healthcare system or hospital likely has well-documented approaches to care based on research and science.

All that said, you still need to find the medical team that you feel most comfortable around. You need to trust them. You need to be able to ask the questions you need to ask, AND you need to be able to understand clearly what they tell you. They should listen to you, and they shouldn't dismiss your concerns. If you have a worry, they should address it and not brush it aside. Just because your primary care doctor recommended a certain oncologist or surgeon, doesn't mean you have to stay with them.

It's okay to get a second opinion. Or a third opinion. Keep looking until you're happy.

When I was diagnosed with breast cancer, I was referred to a breast surgeon in my healthcare network. As I sat in her waiting room with my husband, ten minutes ticked by. Then twenty. Then thirty. We kept asking the receptionist whether we'd be next. She said we would be.

Then, another patient came in as we were asking about how much longer it would be.

That patient sighed and said, "She's always late. I haven't even had surgery yet, and she's been late to every appointment."

At forty-five minutes past our scheduled appointment time, she finally saw us.

Now, sometimes, I, myself, run late. I also understand that surgeons can be late because of events outside their control: surgeries that run longer than expected, for instance. But let me tell you, waiting forty-five minutes in a beige and pink waiting room does NOTHING for one's mental health, when getting a consultation on whether or not I cut my boobs off is frankly already nerve-wracking enough.

Also, if this was how she ran her office, how did she run her OR? Would I be knocked out on the table for an hour before she finally managed to show up?

Look, I know doctors are late for many reasons. Sometimes it's because they might be taking longer with a patient who has more questions. I also know that healthcare networks often pressure doctors to squeeze in as many patients as they can in a short amount of time. There are a lot of reasons, and maybe a doctor being late doesn't bother you as it bothers me, and that's fine. But for me, the extra minutes in that waiting room just amped up my already anxious self.

When I finally did get into see her, she gave me the Giant Scary Phonebook of Cancer, and while I did appreciate that, she also seemed to hedge. A lot.

She told me maybe I wouldn't need a mastectomy, which felt wrong to me. I'd seen the mammogram, and the problem areas looked like a constellation of stars across most of my left breast. I didn't even understand how they'd manage a lumpectomy across that much area. What would I be left with? A Pac Man boob, with a mouth carved out? No, thank you.

Also, she kind of hurried us through the appointment, even though *she* was the one who was late.

And, she even said, maybe I should see the oncologist because there's certain kinds of chemo where maybe I wouldn't even need surgery at all! Or. . . actually, maybe I should just get in a mental state for a mastectomy. Might be that too. Huh?

Then, we went to see the oncologist, the one that asked about my health. And he said, *Oh, I'd definitely need surgery. There was no way out of that. Chemo wasn't going to solve this problem on its own, and while he wasn't a surgeon, he felt like a mastectomy is probably what would be required.*

I went to see another surgeon.

This doctor was right on time. She also gave me a Terrifying Phonebook of information—this one branded with a different medical group—and she was blunt.

There's no way a lumpectomy would work. I'd need a mastectomy, and my choice was single or double.

The truth was hard.

But it was also what I needed.

Now, maybe you want a doctor who soft-pedals the bad news and lets you cling to unrealistic hope for a few weeks. Not me. Give it to me straight. Don't pull punches. I need to know what I'm dealing with. I'm not one of those people who deliberately avoids all bad news ever. I want to know.

And that second surgeon, she let me get dressed, sat with me in that windowless room, and answered every one of my questions—and I had many. The appointment was an hour, and I didn't feel rushed, which was good because I went in and out of the white room and had to repeat my questions sometimes to hear the same answers. The doctor wasn't rushed because clearly, for new patients, she scheduled the proper amount of time and didn't run late.

After talking with her, I felt like I better understood what was in front of me. I understood that the path wasn't going to be easy, but at least there was a realistic path. It had a mastectomy or double mastectomy in it, but at the same time, my doctor told me my prognosis was excellent.

And I believe her because she shared the bad news with me.

Women of color, you'll have to advocate harder and louder for yourselves.

Our medical system is flawed and it's bigoted. Black women have a 4% lower rate of breast cancer than white women, but a 40% higher chance of dying from breast cancer.

That is not a fucking typo.

They're less likely to get it in the first place, but way more likely to die of it.[30]

So are Alaskan and Native American women.

Hispanic women? They die at lesser rates than Black women but higher rates than white women.

Asian women, (like me), have a slightly lower death rate than white women. But, fun fact, Asian women had the fastest increase in breast cancer cases among all racial groups, a contest none of us wanted to win.[31]

Many women of color are more likely to get diagnosed with breast cancer at later stages than white and Asian women, putting them behind the eight ball.[32]

Our society is fundamentally unequal, regardless of the American pat-ourselves-on-the-back, we're-not-racist-and-never-were propaganda machine, okay? Healthcare disparities that exist for maternal care and every other level of care also extend to cancer care, and it's not the fault of the patients. It's the fault of our society.

No surprise then that you'll have to advocate longer and louder for the same care. It's even more important that you find a doctor and medical team who take your concerns seriously, answer your questions, and don't patronize you or explain away your pain.

---

[30] Sandy McDowell, "Breast Cancer Death Rates Are Highest for Black Women—Again," *American Cancer Society*, October 3, 2022.
[31] "American Association for Cancer Research Cancer Disparities Progress Report," 2024.
[32] "What women of color should know about metastatic breast cancer," Medical News Today, February 2024.

It's this. Or that.

We walk into the second oncologist's office. There's a sign on the receptionist's glass window that cautions us to be kind to the staff and not to be belligerent. I wonder who's done this, but then it's not that hard of a stretch. It's an *oncologist's* office. People come here facing all stages of cancer. People are angry. They're terrified. They lash out. They fight the people in front of them instead of the cancer in their bodies. Because they can see the people in front of them. It's easy. Simpler.

But the receptionist is soft-spoken. She's gentle. Kind.

PJ and I don't wait long before the nurse calls us back to the exam room. It's the fifth one I've seen in the last two weeks.

Doctors' offices all seem to have the same thing: exam table, a little small side table with computer screen, a rolling stool that stows beneath the table, and a sink that's bone dry because most caregivers opt for the pump dispenser of hand sanitizer fixed to the wall by the door.

This exam room has interesting green marble and diamond-shaped tile above the sink. A little splash of color in the room that's otherwise white with natural wood cabinets and plain handles. The tile is surprising because it's not neutral. I wonder about the contractor, designer, or builder who picked it. Desperate to give a little something. Maybe green for luck, since this is one of a dozen rooms in the Cancer Center.

"I'm just going to take your blood pressure," the nurse says. I almost flinch because I know the reading will be bad.

I offer my arm. She takes the reading and gives me a supportive smile. "Feeling a little nervous?"

"Yeah," I admit. I'm not the calmest sitting here. My knee bobs up and down with nerves. My body wants to bolt. Because who wants this bad news? I want it. I need it. But I fear it at the same time.

"I thought so. It's okay. People usually are." She smiles again. I like her. "It's okay. And, look, we—the nurses—we'll get to know you. If you do have to come back, or if you have more treatments here, we'll all get to know you. You won't be alone."

And you know what? She was 100% right. I did come back. The nurses DID get to know me. One even came to one of my book signings.

In this moment, this first visit, I'm so grateful for that kindness. I know I'm not alone. I've got PJ. I've got my amazing family and friends, but at times like these, I'm stupidly grateful for kindness from medical professionals. I write romance novels for a living. So what? These people save lives. And this nurse is doing it kindly. With grace and a smile. She gives me the permission I didn't even know I needed to have high blood pressure.

The nurse leaves us, promising the doctor will be in soon.

The oncologist knocks and then rushes in, thick dark curls, lush, umber skin flawless, as she shakes my hand. She's young to me, but everyone under the age of 45 looks young to me.

When I was thirty, kids in college started looking like kids in high school. Now, at fifty, thirty-year-olds look like babies. PJ squeezes my hand. He's sitting by my side because he's already told me that I can't keep him away from any doctor's appointment.

She hits the hand sanitizer pump, rubs her hands, and reaches out to shake mine, still wet.

"Sorry about the sanitizer," she says and shrugs.

"You don't have to apologize about being extra clean," I joke, and she smiles.

She settles into the computer, pulls up my chart, and then sets the expectations. "So, we know some things, but not everything. I'm going to get into the details soon, but just wanted you to know that there are still questions."

I know. I have all of them.

She asks me about all the tests I've had: the mammograms, the biopsy, the MRI. She confirms everything that's happened up to now. She tells me what I already know:

Intraductal cancer.

Microinvasive cancer into the breast tissue.

The MRI found a suspicious lymph node.

It also found a cyst on my liver. Which is probably just normal, but we want an MRI to be sure, because everything now is sus. Yes, that's right. They found a cyst on my liver during the MRI, and now they want another MRI.

"Let me just see if I can print this, and..." She hits a few keys on her keyboard. "I don't know if we'll be able to get a print-out, but..."

I'm kind of relieved that doctor's offices have to fight printers, too. At my house, they never work when needed, especially when school papers are due for the kids. They've fought the good fight against printers before.

She leaves, and then returns, empty-handed, with an apologetic shrug. And then she starts talking. There are a lot of Big Words. Because there are always Big Words.

As she's telling us how cancer works. She taps at the screen, showing me three versions of a milk duct: one with just a few cancer cells in it. Bar's got people but it's not crowded. Then, the second, teaming with cancer cells. This bar just got hot and crowded, and nobody can get a drink at the bar. Even if they can, the bartender just ran out of Jager and Fireball.

Then, the third picture, some of the patrons are saying, "Fuck this," and leaving. To find a place to drink that's not hot and sweaty and out of shots. Or, maybe some other posse is talking shit, and they get into a shoving match and everyone is kicked out by the bouncers. Whatever the case, the second those cells spring themselves, the second they start bar hopping, then those bitches are invasive cancer.

"Because you've had microinvasions"—a few bitches left the bar and decided to take their drama down the street—"You're Stage One. But, what we don't know is how aggressive they are."

Right. Are they just fun drunks or angry drunks? Have they punched a cop yet? How bad is this night going to get? This is what I need to know.

A soft knock comes on the door, and the nurse comes in with the printout. The doctor takes it and then flips it over to scribble my options. I'm glad she's writing this down because I know the very second I walk out of this door, I'm going to forget every word.

Option One: the cancer is mostly contained to the ducts. The Jager hasn't run out, and there's still room on the dance floor. Only a few disgruntled bitches left because those are the dramatic ones that make it all about them. When they drink, they pick a fight about that time you went to Cabo without them, even though it was a *work trip* and your boss was watching those hotel receipts like a hawk and would've known if you'd brought a prohibited plus one. You keep these friends around because they're always up for a drink (even though any chance they get they'll stick you with the bill). So, the couple of high maintenance friends are just hanging on the curb, drunk, trying to call an Uber that's yet to arrive.

Treatment for that? Surgery. Maybe no radiation even. No chemo. You cut out those dramatic bitches before their implanted asses hit the backseat of that rideshare.

We shut down the party before the cops were called. Yay, us.

Option Two: the Jager ran out, the DJ sucks, and most people have flooded out to the sidewalk. They don't even wait for an Uber. They just stumble down the block, across the street, everywhere. The cops have the blue and red lights flashing. They shout from their patrol cars, telling people to go home, but they're not listening. Bitches are puking on sidewalks, stumbling into Ubers, demanding to go to the expensive champagne bar, the one with $600 bottles. They're texting "you up?" to their most toxic of exes. They're making ALL THE MISTAKES.

Depending on how many bitches got how far, and whether someone spit on the window of the police car or not, this could be Stage Two or Stage Two B.

This could mean chemo then surgery. Or surgery then chemo. It means nobody is going home tonight until all the bitches are round up, contained at home, not at an ex's or in jail.

This is the worst Choose Your Own Adventure book of all time.

Also – this was the cancer I was facing. Others need hormonal treatments. Everybody is unique, okay?

But what I kept feeling during all this, was the moving target.

First, it was so early it was stage zero. Maybe one at most.

Now, I'm all the way up to 2b, maybe, or worse?

Can we stop adding to this tally, please? Can I hold here? I don't want more. I don't want any more stages. I'm not a caterpillar.

"I still think, the best course is likely to be surgery. We'll do the pathology and then we'll know what we're dealing with."

Is this a mild girls' night where the worst we do is dance on a table? Or is this the kind of night where someone leaves a phone, a wallet, and at least one shoe in an Uber, and another pukes, so the driver skids to a stop and kicks us all off on an exit ramp of the expressway? We get into a crying, screaming match with the driver and each other, and then the fire department shows up with puke bags and judgment. Then the state police are called after that one friend tries to dash across the freeway. She's arrested for throwing her one remaining shoe at a trooper. Are we mildly hungover or drunk and disorderly?

"We probably won't know for sure until a week after surgery," the doctor tells me. "They're like weeds," she tells me.

You can be skeptical of traditional medicine as well. That's your right.

Now, my mom is skeptical of the medical community. She hasn't actually gone to the doctor in years, and I think it's because she was married to my dad (a surgeon) for twenty-five years before they got divorced. The shine of the medical establishment, let's just say, wore off for her. Her parents also hated doctors, so maybe it's a learned thing.

Who knows?

Anyway, the point is:—if you don't want to go to a doctor and get traditional treatment, that's your right.

Cancer doesn't get to decide your care, but neither does your doctor.

This is YOUR journey.

Now, for the record, I chose traditional medicine. I trust science (see Dad as doctor), and I went with the treatment backed by dozens of studies. In my research, traditional medicine was most likely to save my life.

But that was my journey.

Not yours.

I would—and never will—tell anyone how to treat their cancer.

There's no easy treatment. There's no easy way out, no matter which path you choose.

I decided to go all in with traditional medicine—because I wanted to fight this as hard as I could, and they had the most powerful weapons, with definitive, statistical research, to back it up. Traditional medicine is also the scariest route—it requires a scalpel, poisonous chemotherapy chemicals, and scarring radiation—but it also produces results.

I trust science and research, but I don't expect it to be infallible. It changes all the time, and while some people feel that's bad, I think it's a good thing because that means we learn more. The more we discover, the better treatments can get. I also accept that treatment isn't perfect. It might never be perfect. But these are the best weapons we have right now, and I am just not the kind of person to bring organic kale to a gunfight.

All that said, this is a JUDGMENT-FREE ZONE. If you opt to switch your diet to only turmeric quinoa and that you're going to meditate the cancer away, that's YOUR choice. I would never in a million years judge anyone for any decision they made regarding treatment. Everyone has lines inside them they do not want to cross.

Some women will fight to keep their breasts, no matter what. Others refuse to have chemicals in their body. I would never suggest that you second-guess your beliefs. Every breast cancer patient must live with their decisions—the treatments they decide to get, and no one can walk in their shoes.

We are the ones who have to live with our decisions, so they have to be OURS.

It's okay to do your own research, just don't let it rule your life.

Look, you already know what Web MD is going to tell you. You've got a death sentence. I mean, we've already looked up that "weird pain in my side" and discovered in a single google search we're at death's door.

Now that you have a diagnosis, you'll find an avalanche of terrifying info online. It's okay to dig deep.

Just don't live in that rabbit hole.

Some people deal with stress by finding out as much information as possible, from as many sources as possible, and then try to exorcise their fear demons with spreadsheets and links and lists of experimental medicines.

If this is your way of coping, fine.

Just don't let it become an obsession. It's easy to be consumed by fact-finding and research, but there's SO MUCH out there, and unless you're an oncologist yourself, much of it is hard to truly understand.

Avengers, Assemble!

"You're going to assemble your team. Your doctors. Your surgeons," my counselor tells me. "They're going to be the *best* team. *Your* team. The people you feel comfortable with. The people you trust."

I nod.

"And you're going to lean on this team."

I already have been. The nurse navigators, the breast surgeon, the plastic surgeon, the oncologist, the geneticist, the physical therapist, the dietician, the radiologists, the doctors who performed the biopsies, everyone.

"Yes, I have been. Already." I didn't like doing it, I'll admit. Leaning on others wasn't something I ever really am *comfortable* doing.

"It doesn't make you any less superwoman," she tells me. "Even she needed help from her team. Even superheroes need help sometimes."

Take ownership of your care.

While I hated leaning on people, ironically, I never really second-guessed my healthcare treatment before. I trusted the people in white coats. Maybe it's because my dad was a doctor, or that I always thought the kids in math and science who did well *had* to be smarter than me (math was never my strong suit). I dutifully showed up for annual physicals and ob/gyn exams, and then whatever they told me, I pretty much did. Did I have a sinus infection? Take the antibiotics. Was my vitamin D level low? Okay, take supplements.

This relationship didn't require me to be very vigilant or involved. I didn't even have to like my doctors *that* much—who cared when I saw them for an hour every year?

Breast cancer is a different beast. I encourage you to ask questions, to be difficult sometimes, and not to follow along blindly without knowing what it is you're getting into. This doesn't mean to resist treatment. What I'm saying is that you need to understand it, and not just be okay with it, be all in with it. Do not offer knee-jerk compliance.

We—especially us women—are trained from a very young age to be compliant.[33]

In *Defy* by Dr. Sunita Sah, she delves into all the ways we're programmed to believe that being a "good" child means obeying and being "bad" means defying authority—even when that authority is bad. She delves into the substantial research that shows that, even when people are asked to do something they think is wrong, the urge to comply is so strong that they often do it, even if they feel bad. Our social programming to go along, even when we don't want to, often explains mind-boggling situations. Nazi officers that "just followed orders" at death camps during the Holocaust. Or the officers standing by and doing nothing as George Floyd was murdered by another police officer in Minneapolis. Dr. Sah argues that as much as we'd like to believe we'd be different—we'd speak out or resist – that many of us would ALSO simply fall back on social programming. We'd feel badly about it, but we'd comply.

---

[33] Sunita Sah, MD. *Defy: The Power of No in a World That Demands Yes*, Random House, January 14, 2025.

We are compliant all the time to avoid social awkwardness, even when we'd rather say no. Dr. Sah even discussed an incident in her own personal life where she was pressured to get an CT scan she didn't need, and despite knowing she didn't need it, she went along with it anyway. In her book, she underscores the difference between compliance and consent. Compliance is going along, even when we have reservations, we feel it's wrong, or it goes against our core values. Consent is our true yes—our hell, yes—if you will. Consent is active. Compliance is passive. It's up to us to figure out our True Yes and our True No, and that requires that we lean into uncomfortable feelings (are we saying yes because we truly mean yes or are we just bowing to social pressure?).

Dr. Sah suggests that one way we can avoid knee-jerk compliance—especially when we feel uncomfortable—is to NOT make a decision right there.

So, if your oncologist says, "You must do chemo. We'll schedule you next week," it's perfectly acceptable to say, "Wait. I need some time to think about this."

You're not saying "no." You're saying "maybe" and "maybe" is a LOT easier to say than "no" in some of these situations. I say "maybe" all the time to my kids, and this usually means no (they've caught on and now say, "Maybe means 'no', Mom!").

And I cannot stress this enough: You can always say MAYBE. You can ALWAYS say, "I need a minute." You can ALWAYS call a time-out. Sometimes, when you're in a room filled with white coats, you don't feel like you can say no. But you can ALWAYS say no. You can absolutely say maybe.

This is your body and your life; you can hit pause ANY DAMN TIME YOU FEEL LIKE IT.

Okay?

You are giving your consent to be treated. And you can revoke it at any time.

Think of it as you in the bedroom with a lover. Just because you agreed to be there in the first place, it doesn't mean that you ALSO agreed to hang from the ceiling upside down with a ball gag in your mouth. Your consent is required at every step and every stage, and even if you gave it at the start, YOU, my friend, can revoke it at any time. You can tell your oncologist mid-treatment that you don't like the treatment. You can hit the pause button if you need to. And knowing that you CAN hit the pause button will fill you up with courage. You know why?

Because you're in control, that's why.

You can get off this ride any time you want.

My grandfather defied the medical community at the end of his life.

My mother's father possessed a faulty heart valve. It caused him pain and shortness of breath, and his cardiologist said he needed heart surgery. My grandfather—in his mid-seventies—didn't want heart surgery. He hated hospitals and doctors in general. He didn't want to spend a week in the hospital. The cardiologist told him with the surgery he'd live, and without it, he'd die. Maybe this year, maybe next, but he'd die.

My grandfather's answer? "I've lived long enough."

He opted not to get the surgery. He moved in with my mother, who cared for him, and he spent the time he had left doing what he loved (usually playing slot machines) and died within two years.

But that was his decision.

This was the first time in my life I'd heard of someone declining treatment. It left a powerful impression on me because I'd never in my life considered *not* getting treatment, especially if it were life-saving treatment, but my grandfather said no.

Now, I wasn't about to decline life-saving surgery. I went the opposite route. He was in his mid-seventies. I'm 51. His grandchildren were long grown. My children weren't yet through high school.

I went scorched earth on my cancer because I might be a pacifist, but if you mess with me, I'm going to mess with you.

The whole point is YOUR body, your life, your choice.

So, do not sleepwalk through your care. I encourage you to actually look for doctors you LIKE, vibe with, and trust because you're literally entrusting them with your LIFE.

What does taking ownership of your care look like? Like this:

- **Ask questions.** Make sure you understand what they're telling you. Don't skip the details. Understand what's happening—both inside your body and with the treatments they want to give you.
- **Find doctors you're comfortable with and trust.** Your doctor should be a vibe—a vibe you LIKE. If you hate your doctor, this is going to be a long road.
- **Research your care team.** Do they have good reviews? Bad reviews?
- **Don't always just go with the medical group or care center closest to you.** We're built to love convenience, but you might find that a much nicer, newer, friendlier care center (still in your network, of course) is a forty-minute drive instead of a four-minute drive. Maybe the extra time is worth it for better care.
- **Make sure you understand what it all costs and what's your share.** We'll get into the weeds on this in "Chapter Eleven: Soul Crushing Debt," but as you're choosing your care team, it's also important you understand what your insurance will and won't pay. Most doctors won't even do surgery unless it's pre-

approved by your health insurance. But if no one is talking about your insurance, make sure you ask. Trying to understand your portion of costs (as much as you can in our wonky healthcare system where for some reason the cost of everything is a secret) the better off you'll be.

- **When doctors recommend a course of treatment, make sure inside you, you feel a "Hell, yes!" and not a "I guess I need to go along with this because they said so, but I feel weird about it."** Don't comply just because you feel you should. Say "maybe" or say "I'll think about it," so that you can find time to dig deep and get to how you REALLY feel about it. I'm not saying run from care because you're scared. We're all scared because it's all terrifying, but if deep within you, you know you need to throw everything and the at the kitchen sink at caner, then *do it.*

Assemble Your Own Team of Avengers

You can't do this alone. I mean, you can try, but I wouldn't operate on myself.

So.

You'll need a team.

May I suggest the most bad-ass team of Avengers ever that will kick cancer's ass? You'll want them to send cancer back to hell where it belongs.

You'll need an Iron Man, a Captain Marvel, a Captain America, a Thor, a Spiderman, and a Black Widow. You'll need them all.

You'll need to trust your team.

Remember, Cancer is the Enemy.

Not the doctors. Not your spouse. Not your kids.

Cancer is the enemy.

Cancer will try to fool you. It will try to misdirect your anger to someone who doesn't deserve it, like the nurse drawing your blood, the MRI tech trying to get the IV in, or the doctor who says you need ANOTHER biopsy (my God, how many times you can poke my lymph nodes via armpit needles? Are you all sick sadists?!). Cancer will gladly let you believe you're really angry at your kid who talks back to you or your spouse who forgets to unload the dishwasher.

But they're not who you're mad at.

You're mad at cancer.

Cancer is the enemy.

I once had a nurse navigator (that's the person in charge of coordinating your care) call me to reschedule a surgeon's visit. She told me the news quickly as if she were flinching on the other line, waiting for me to explode. When I didn't, and I was just a normal person who understood that sometimes surgeons got sick because they're human, that waiting another two days wouldn't, actually, kill me, she melted into a pool of relief.

"Oh, my goodness, you're so amazing," she gushed. "I just got off the phone with someone who. . ." She hesitated, trauma clear in her voice. "Well, who didn't take it so well."

"You're just doing your job," I told her. "Cancer is the enemy. I know who I'm really fighting."

I *knew* who I was the angriest at in all the world. It wasn't the doctor who got me sick. Or the nurse who had to reschedule patients. It was the fucking cancer trying to kill me.

This nurse navigator was so relieved and grateful to be talking to a calm human that she also sent me a thank-you note in My Chart. Imagine being this poor nurse. She got into medicine in the first place to help people, and she thought *what better place to do that than cancer patients who need my help the most of all?* And then she gets into her work only to discover that most of the cancer patients hate on her all day. They scream and yell and call her names, all because she's just trying to *help them live*. And all because they hadn't handled their fear (see Chapter Two: Face Your Fear) or because they were letting their inner toddler throw tantrums of a lifetime (Chapter Ten: The Only Way Is Through).

Y'all—you don't have to be a fucking gazelle through this process (Chapter Nineteen: You Don't Have to Be a Gazelle), but you DO need to treat other humans that are honestly trying to help you with just decent courtesy. Yes, you're having the worst time of your life, but berating innocent people will only make you feel bad about yourself. So don't be your own kryptonite.

Did you know that 17.5% of registered nurses leave their profession in the first year, and more than a third leave by the end of year two?[34]

All you have to be is a reasonably polite human, and you'll maybe help a nurse remember why he or she got into this profession to begin with.

You're irritable and annoyed and frustrated. . . because of CANCER.

The doctors and nurses will tell you things you don't want to hear. But they are TRYING TO HELP YOU. (Unless they're terrible doctors—which, we've been over this, you don't have to continue to see them).

Your coworkers will be their annoying selves, but is it really that "per my last email" making you want to murder them? Or is it cancer?

Your spouse, friends, or relatives won't be as supportive as you like, *when* you like, but you're not really mad at them, are you?

---

[34] Ellen Rice Tichich, MFA, MSN, RN-BC, "Recruitment and Retention Efforts Address Oncology Nursing Shortage," *Oncology Nursing News*, March 2019.

Cancer would LOVE it if you shout at them, if you blame them, if you push them away. Because then you forget who the real enemy is. Then you forget who you're fighting.

You're fighting cancer. Don't let it distract you.

If you're too busy fighting all the people trying to help you, then you'll forget who the real enemy is.

It's cancer you want to throttle, so don't take it out on everyone else.

Cancer is the enemy.

Pep talk #7:

Hey, there. Feeling frustrated by your caregivers and our healthcare system in general? Feeling let down by your insurance? Want to burn the whole system down? I feel you. I've been there. Are you a woman of color feeling lost in the shuffle?

Don't give up hope. Keep looking for a doctor that really sees and hears you, one that clicks with you. Don't settle for the first referral you get if that person rubs you the wrong way. This is your team of Avengers, your superheroes to help you, and you should believe in them 100%. You don't have to be polite and nice and considerate to a surgeon you don't like.

Ghost the hell out of them. That's fine.

You will find caregivers who have your back. Go to battle with the best of the best.

You're about to have the fight of your life, so make sure your fellow soldiers in the trenches have your back.

Chapter Eight

Your Imagination Is (Almost) Always Worse Than Reality

"We suffer more in our imagination than in reality."

—Seneca

I'm a romance novelist. I have a pretty damn good imagination. So when the doctors tell me what treatment they think I should have, my imagination goes to the worst possible scenarios. When there's this looming monster of breast cancer, but no real understanding of how to kill it, that stuff is terrifying. The treatments for me sometimes felt scarier than the cancer itself.

For me, doctors laid out a whole lot of scary treatments on the table, and with every single one, there seemed to be something horrible attached. Your own imagination (and the Worst Phonebook of All Time) can just fuel the fear if you go down the chemo road, or the surgery road, or the radiation road, or all three. I started expecting the worst.

You might be here, too. You might be fearing the worst.

And you know what? It might be the worst.

Or it might not.

Most of the time, our imaginations bring forth the worst possible scenarios to try to scare us to death, but reality might not be what we feared. Actually, it'll probably be something completely different.

Let's break down how our imaginations scare us to death. Let's start with pain.

I'm scared of pain.

I'll be the first to admit this.

I am not one of those people who embraces BDSM and loves a good whack. I hate pain. HATE it. Fear it. Loathe it. Run from it. While I couldn't wait to have kids, I also dreaded the birth of both my children because I feared pain on a deep, visceral level. I never even entertained the thought of having a birth without an epidural. Nope. No, thank you. Only your *best* drugs for me, thank you very much. Top shelf, not rail, please, bartender.

If you don't fear pain, man, I want to live in *your* head for a while. What's it like to feel invincible?

The thing is, I fear pain because I don't like it, but also because I worry that I'll do something foolish or cowardly or embarrassing while in the throes of pain. I don't know why I worry about this. It doesn't make sense to worry about this at the same level as I worry about actually feeling pain, but I do.

Maybe it's a Gen X thing, like you're not supposed to show fear of pain on the playground or you'll be devoured. Fall off the rusted death trap of a merry-go-round? Better not cry unless you're a first grader. Anything older than that, and you'll be made fun of relentlessly for the rest of your days in elementary school.

Maybe it was all that good old-fashioned bullying of the '80s. I don't know.

But whatever it is, I fear pain and how it will make me act, so I try to avoid it at all costs. Most reasonable people do. Do you know what most people will do with just *the threat* of pain? They will do almost anything. They will hand over their wallets and their money. They will beg or plead.

Every cancer treatment comes with a side of pain and discomfort.

No matter where I looked, each treatment—surgery or chemo or radiation—came with pain.

And in my imagination, this pain was all-encompassing, mind-numbing, mind-altering pain. That's because I've got a good imagination, and imagination is trying to *keep us alive*. If my imagination said, "Oh, I bet it's really not that bad to get bitten by a shark" then I might go ahead and swim in the ocean at dusk or dawn, ignoring the all the fins sticking out of the water with zero fear. But my brain imagines that shit would be fucking awful, for good reason. It's trying to help me avoid doing something dumb like put my head in an alligator's mouth.

But, I'll let you in on a little secret. The pain in our imagination is likely greater than the pain in real life (except, I'll tell you, for childbirth. Man, that shit lives UP to the hype. For my second daughter, I got an epidural too late. I had the baby 100% before any of the meds kicked in, and I would've sworn to you that I died and left my body.). The point I'm trying to make is that the level of pain you imagine isn't the same level as pain in real life. The pain and discomfort you're likely going to face from cancer treatments can be:

a) Mostly managed by drugs

b) Isn't nonstop—without breaks

c) Again, not as bad—or—at the very least—different than what you fear.

You'll be knocked out for the very worst of the pain.

I imagined that recovering from having both my breasts lopped off would be worse than any other cut or wound I'd ever had.

I imagined this in my mind in chilling detail. It didn't help that I really hate the idea of being stabbed. With pretty much anything—needles, knives, anything really. I don't want to be stabbed. Or cut. Or sliced. I think I'm in the majority of people here when I say the idea of getting jabbed with anything is horrible. Even if it is an award-winning surgeon with a scalpel. I still don't like being sliced into, thank you very much. I am not a Thanksgiving turkey.

I feared the surgery. I feared it so much that, despite all the meditating and prepping for surgery, when they wheeled me in on the gurney and I saw those fucking giant lights from *Gray's Anatomy* hanging from the ceiling, I felt a panic attack coming on. Thank God for the anesthesiologist who just turned up the juice in my IV and then I was out. No counting, no nothing. Just flat OUT.

What I feared was the idea of being cut—of being sawed on—when I was awake. But, I wasn't awake. I was completely out. I came to, bandaged and hopped up on drugs, having barely felt a thing. Also, when they took my boobs, they also took almost every nerve ending in the place, so I actually didn't have many pain receptors at all.

I mean, I had some. The cuts were sore. They hurt. My inner chest wall—the muscles there—were bruised and sore. But it wasn't debilitating. And it wasn't CONSTANT pain, either. Sometimes, when I lay very still, in certain positions, I didn't have much pain at all.

I could *control* the pain a little—by how I moved, how I laid down, and what painkillers I took.

You will have some control over your pain.

While I managed my pain after surgery, I came to realize that maybe it wasn't the pain I feared so much as the thought of being out of control. That the pain would drive me, and I'd be along for the ride, that I'd have no levers to pull, no pedals to press.

But I had things I could do. I could use pillows to prop myself up in a certain way. I could take painkillers. I could use CBD. Or the opioids I'd been prescribed. If the pain got worse, I could reach out to my doctor and ask for solutions. I wasn't just a victim to pain, a hapless bystander to my life. I had agency.

That's what we FORGET to imagine when we're painting a picture in our minds of our worst-case scenario. We fail to remember that WE can do things to help ourselves. That the pain won't be so overwhelming all the time that we won't be able to fight it.

Hell, sometimes, you're going to sleep. And you won't feel it then.

And even better, the pain will get less and less.

For me, for each day that passed, the pain got a little less. So I knew that every new day would dawn and I'd be a little bit better, a little bit stronger, with a little less hurting. Each day I could walk a little farther. Each day I was a little less tired, a little less fatigued.

We deal with pain in our daily lives all the time.

You, my friend, likely deal with a regular onslaught of aches and pains because, if you're not eighteen, you're probably walking around in a body that gets sore. Randomly. Maybe even for no reason. I once threw my back out, I swear, *from sleeping.*

We deal with the thud of background pain all the time. Period cramps. Sore muscles. Pulled muscles. Paper cuts. A twisted ankle. Wonky knee. Headaches. Pain is actually a regular part of life. When you start to think about pain that way, you realize it's no stranger to you. It pops up all the time. Do we melt into a puddle when we get a headache? No, we don't. We pop an aspirin and move on. We trudge through all kinds of discomforts as women (stilettos, tight pants, shaping underwear, fake eyelashes), and we do it with a smile.

The pain you'll feel from treatments or surgery will likely be worse, sure, but it won't be *off the charts* worse.

Remember that you've got a whole lifetime of dealing and managing with pain.

The only thing worse than pain? Embarrassment.

Okay, so the pain might not be that bad. And it might be manageable.

But what about feeling embarrassed?

Let's talk about it.

Let's talk about feeling embarrassed.

I hate to feel embarrassed. I think I'd *rather* feel physical pain than embarrassment.

I'm not alone in this, either. In colonial days, when the Puritans would lock up adulterers and other offenders in the town square in the stockades so that their neighbors could jeer at them and throw rotten cabbages or tomatoes at them for a day or two, the punishment was so dreaded that sometimes people would choose death or a severe beating to avoid it.[35]

We're hard-wired to want to avoid that kind of humiliation because embarrassment and humiliation threaten our position in the tribe, and we all fear excommunication because, historically, rejection from the group meant certain death.

Let's be honest—the idea of getting chemo pumped into your veins and losing your hair or having radiation voluntarily blasted at your chest—is terrifying but it's also embarrassing. The first time I walked into a restaurant with a scarf covering my bald-ass head during chemo treatment, I was certain everyone was judging me, talking about me, wondering what

---

[35] Jon Ronson, *So You've Been Publicly Shamed,* 2016.

was wrong with me. It was exactly the kind of attention I never asked for and never wanted.

And I will be lying to you if I didn't mention I worried about that. About being embarrassed. About looking strange. About being a freak. About people pointing and whispering.

And I didn't just worry about what I looked like to perfect strangers, either. I spent a considerable amount of time worried about making a fool of myself in front of medical personnel. Why? I don't know. Maybe it was because I flopped half-naked onto that MRI table early on in this process, but I did NOT want to be the "you won't believe this patient" story from *any* of my nurses. I had my dignity and my pride, and I didn't want to give those up. In my imagination, getting these treatments for cancer—hell, even having cancer at all—was a little embarrassing.

But here's the thing about embarrassment.

Most of the things we're embarrassed about—other people don't even notice, or if they do, they don't care. And if they do care, it's whole lot less than we think. We spend a lot of time worried about what other people think, but most of the time, they're not even thinking about us.

This is what psychologists refer to as the Spotlight Effect. Say you stain your shirt. Suddenly, you believe that everyone has noticed your stained shirt and has judged you for it. This is the Spotlight Effect. We believe we—and our mistakes—are on display on stage in a spotlight.[36]

Don't believe that people really don't care about your stained shirt or your bald head?

Think about this: when you're in public, how often are you actively judging other people, and how often are you just thinking about your life and the things you need to get done?

---

[36] Aditi Subramaniam, Ph.D, "All Eyes on Us: The Spotlight Effect – How a psychological bias causes us to overestimate how much people notice us," *Psychology Today*, June 20, 2022.

Say you're at the grocery store and you see someone who's bald and sickly. Do you really spend a lot of time thinking about them? Or are you thinking about your grocery list and how you have to get home and cook dinner? Most of the time do you just do a pity and pivot in your own head? Sure you do.

Right. See?

Everyone you meet isn't in the spotlight, and yet you feel you're special? No. Stop being an egomaniac, okay? People aren't noticing you as much as you think. And that's a good thing.

You have control.

Also, even if people judge us—so what? The only way you can actually be embarrassed is to care what other people think.

You, warrior, have cancer. And you may not look ready for a close-up because you don't have eyebrows or eyelashes, but the fact is you're a bad-ass motherfucker who is kicking cancer's ass, and that's more beautiful than waist-length tresses. And even so, there are wigs, fake eyelashes, and even temporary tattooed eyebrows. You can 100% fake it till you make it.

Yes, people will look at you when you walk in bald—or with a scarf on your head or the poorly fitted wig—but you are still YOU. You are funny or you're smart or you're caring and kind—whatever makes you uniquely you is still there.

And there's no reason to be embarrassed because you're in the fight of your life.

And—again—in your imagination, you're just embarrassed with no recourse. But in reality? You have control over your embarrassment. You get to decide if you're really embarrassed or not. You get to hang with people who make you feel strong, not humiliated. You get to go to places that celebrate you, not tear you down.

Or if you're really feeling low, you can stay home. You can be comfy on the couch. You don't have to parade yourself in public if you don't feel like it.

You get to control situations that make you feel more or less embarrassed.

Embarrassment also isn't a permanent state of mind. It's temporary. It comes and goes. You might feel a little embarrassed about that wig you bought on Amazon. Then don't wear it. Or get a new one. There are ways we can pivot and adapt to our circumstances to make them more comfortable.

Hell, after I finished immunotherapy, I broke out with a bacterial staph infection. ON MY FACE. It was SO fucking embarrassing.

The oncology nurse (my least favorite one in the practice—look, they can't all be angels) told me this was the kind of infection little kids get. "Have you been hanging out with little kids?" she scoffed.

Only later did I feel vindicated by my dermatologist. "This is in the literature," she assured me. "This is a documented side effect."

And this wasn't the first time I'd had something embarrassing on my face. The chemo had caused a horrific outbreak of acne several times, and I needed prescription Benzoyl Peroxide to knock it out. But the bacterial infection? Way, way worse. It hurt and it itched, and even worse than that, it oozed yellow goo.

Sorry. Gross, I know. Think of how the woman sitting next to me on the plane from LAX to O'Hare felt. I'd just gone to visit relatives when the worst of the infection kicked in. And that wasn't even an obviously explainable thing like a scarf over a bald head. It was just weird and gross. Antibiotics knocked it out, but for a few days, I did not want to show my face anywhere. And I didn't.

And that's okay. You DO have some control over that (unless you have a flight you can't cancel). But even then—so what? When was I ever going to see those passengers again? Never.

Our imaginations leave out that part again and again.

Our imaginations just paint the worst possible picture where we have zero agency, can't change a damn thing, and we're stuck.

This isn't how life works.

You can change your mind.

Your imagination will be giving you the worst-case scenario, and it will also lie, telling you that once you start down a path there's no turning back.

This is a lie.

You could start chemo, and then when it becomes unbearable, you can stop. Remember that you are giving consent to treatment and you can revoke it at any time. You can change your mind.

Or maybe ask your doctor to try a different combination of drugs because these are freakin' killing you.

You don't necessarily have to pick a route of treatment only to discover there's no off-ramp. There's almost always an off-ramp. Your doctor may not like it, but there's almost always an off-ramp. There's no off-ramp with surgery, unless you just decide not to do it, but you can always decide NOT to have extra surgeries—reconstruction, for instance.

Your imagination likes to tell you a horror story where you're stuck, have no control over anything, and can't reverse direction, so you better not even TRY to do anything.

That's fear talking. Remember fear from Chapter Two?

Fear talks a good game, but fear is NOT reality.

Fear is the turbulence, not the plane crashing.

Sometimes, you get a break.

When I was getting chemo, I also had to do a book signing. My book was out, and this event had been planned MONTHS in advance. I just didn't feel I could skip it. I was worried about the book signing because it would be two days after a scheduled infusion, and I'd learned that I never knew how I would be feeling two days after. Sometimes, I was fine, but other times, I spent half the day in bed.

So, I was worried. I talked to my doctor about it, told her I was worried, and since I'd picked a doctor who listened to my worries, she said, "Well, we could just skip a round."

Skip one? This had NEVER occurred to me as a possibility. My imagination had told me that once I was on the chemo path there was no changing the calendar, and I'd just be on that horrible ride till it ended. But my doctor said they skip one all the time (like if someone is sick, their blood work is alarming, or any number of reasons). And that skipping one won't hurt the treatment at all.

So. . . I skipped a treatment.

And I felt FUCKING AMAZING for my book signing.

And then I went back to regular treatments with the knowledge that, when chemo stopped, I'd start feeling better RIGHT AWAY.

So, even if you're on a path of treatment, there might be ways to tweak it so you can still live your life. This is why finding your team of Avengers and doctors who listen and work with you is so important (remember Chapter Seven?).

Don't listen to fear, and don't let your imagination convince you that's exactly how it's going to happen because it won't unfold just in that way.

Since when did *anything* happen exactly as you thought since you were diagnosed?

Exactly my point.

Pep talk #8:

Hey, Badass, and you ARE a Badass, did you know that being courageous means you're scared as hell? Yeah, it's the secret that no one tells you.

Brave people are often (almost always) scared shitless. Our imaginations are running wild about just how bad the outcomes are going to be, but we keep putting one foot in front of the other, even though we are 100% positive we're going to fall on our face any second.

You might be obsessing about the worst possible outcomes. Surprise—reality will be different than you imagine. It's probably going to be better than you think. At the very least, it will be different. It won't play out exactly as you fear.

Fear tells you that you have no control, but this is your life, and you do.

Hang in there, Badass.

Keep on going and you might find things aren't as terrible as your feared.

And no matter what, brighter, better days are coming.

Chapter Nine

When Your Body Betrays You—Let's Talk About What We're Really Pissed About

"To me, the thing that is worse than death is betrayal."

—Malcolm X

Cancer wasn't the first time my body tried to kill me.

It also tried to kill me when I was pregnant with my first child.

Let's take a step into the way-back time machine.

I'd always wanted to be a mom and was over the moon when I found out I was pregnant with my first child. I couldn't wait to tell *everyone*, even though I was told to wait until the second trimester, until after the twelfth week. I just. . . could not hold onto that secret. I was overjoyed. It had taken me longer than I thought to get pregnant and every morning I woke up nauseous and I felt the buzz of excitement. I'm going to have a baby! When would my stomach poke out? When would I need stretchy pants? Would I want to know if it's a boy or a girl? I couldn't wait to gallop through all the *firsts* of my first pregnancy.

Then, one morning, I woke up to spotting.

Blood, where there wasn't supposed to be blood. My doctor told me this could be bad, or it could mean nothing, and she'd talk to me the next day at my twelfth week appointment. The spotting stopped, so I figured—we're all good, right? But that's when my doctor couldn't find the baby's heartbeat.

The baby died in utero, at some undetermined point, when I *didn't even know*. Worse, my body never expelled the baby on its own, and now I was at risk of an infection. I'd need a DNC, a procedure that's often done as part of an abortion. Thankfully, medical intervention was legal, so I could get the care I need. In many abortion-ban states, the laws do not consider complications of pregnancy and do not have health of the mother exceptions.

It was the first time I'd felt deep, stinging betrayal by my own body. She couldn't grow the baby I desperately wanted, and she'd been lying to me for days, weeks, or who knows how long. How many mornings now had I woke up with the joy of thinking I was carrying a new life, when there'd been only death inside me? And now she was trying to fucking kill me, too.

All the while, I didn't know.

I slipped into a serious depression. I didn't want to eat, go out, work, or do anything for weeks. The death of my first baby (a girl, by the way, who I named Alexandra) felt bigger than just the loss of a child. It was the death of hope itself—the loss of our future. Grief came at me as grief does—on its own timeline. I spent a long while seeking out self-destructive behaviors because I wanted to punish myself and, most especially, my body. I made one poor decision after another because what did it even matter anyway? My baby died. I might not ever even be able to have one again. Maybe I was broken and defective.

Eventually, I righted the ship. I found my way back to myself. I was fortunate enough to become a mom—twice over. I put this part of my past behind me.

And then two decades later came the cancer diagnosis.

The anger was still fresh.

Anger—fury—roared back to the surface. How quickly I could tap back into that resentment for my own body! You might feel this as well. You might feel like your body betrayed you in the worst possible way. You want to live, but your body wants to die. How is this even possible? How can it *do* this to you? You thought you had a deal, an exclusive relationship: We both want to live. Let's both live. Sure, not forever, but for a decent amount of time, an expected amount of time.

But, really, your breasts are just being selfish. Because cancer cells are just cells that won't die.[37] The reason why cancer is so terrible is that tumors keep growing—and they never die. Other cells in our body—our skin cells, blood cells, pretty much every cell—at some point gets old and dies, and a new, younger cell takes its place. The old cells go out for the good of the whole. That's how we humans work.

But my breast cells? They never wanted to die. And they kept replicating, faster even than normal cells, as they jammed up the works. They were selfish. They wanted to live forever. They wanted to keep on dividing forever, making new copies of themselves, and never die. They wanted to take up all the oxygen—literally—and now they weren't going to self-sacrifice for the greater good. They put themselves over everyone else, and they'd grow and grow and grow forever, squeezing out all the healthy cells, the ones who know when it's their time to go.

Be angry. Let the feelings out. Most importantly, get clear that you ARE furious and you DO feel betrayed. Man, blast those break-up songs. The songs of betrayal will never feel more relevant than now. You have every reason to feel this way. Your body, your most trusted companion all your life, is trying to kill you.

---

[37] Carrie Cowan, Ph.D "How do cancer cells achieve immortality?" *The Jackson Laboratory*, June 28, 2018.

You, too, might have felt betrayed by your body at one time or another. We have high standards, after all, and society has even higher standards (we're all supposed to never age and look like celebrities do at seventy). We're supposed to have certain-sized boobs or ass and spend whatever amount is necessary to always look young and pretty.

But this betrayal, *this* time, feels just so very horrible.

As with any betrayal, the fundamental issue is that you trusted your body to have your back, and it didn't. You expected it to toe the line, that the old cells would die, young ones would take their place, and the cycle would continue. But it didn't. You felt you could lean on it and trust it would live up to its side of the bargain (keeping you both alive), but it didn't.

The trust with your body has been betrayed.

And with this loss of trust comes a feeling of *loss*. You've lost something precious to you. That's really why your emotions are all over the place. You've lost something irreplaceable. How do you ever get it back?

Realize that your mind is the grown-up, and your body is the child.

I was so very angry at myself, at my body, that I wanted to punish it. Sometimes, the pokes and prodding from all those diagnostic tests felt almost good. Like *there*, body, are you happy now? Your stupid antics bring *this* punishment. *This* is what you get for misbehaving. *This* is what you get for breaking the rules.

Honestly, when I hit the treadmill in anger (as I often did), and my knees hurt, or leg muscles felt tired and sore, I thought *you brought this on yourself. Deal with it!*

It took me a long time to realize that my body was basically my inner child. It had no understanding of what it was doing. It didn't know. This seems obvious to a person not in the throes of cancer, but it's hard not to take cancer personally. It just is. With Her 2+ cancer, my immune system fed the cancer, instead of stomping it out, and as far as my body knew, it was simply making cells grow quickly like it had done all its life, with my skin and hair and fingernails, making certain cells grow even faster because *look how efficient I am!*

Once I started feeling like my body was a child and my mind was the grown-up, it helped a lot. It helped me see that my body was a mindless, immature Id, just running around on autopilot, literally with its head cut off. My brain, my consciousness, was the adult in its life, its guardian, the one who was supposed to put up the guardrails but also, most importantly, protect it from itself.

For any of you parents out there, you know that every single toddler on the planet has a death wish. Mine tried to kill themselves a million ways every single day. Electric socket available? They'd try to jam their fingers or, preferably, a fork into it. Sharp glass corner? They'd smack it with their foreheads every time. Busy street? They'd run toward it full speed, without looking, every single time.

Your body is a little like that. It's a child who doesn't understand consequences or basic logic. Your conscious, logical brain does. So, it's up to you to look after your body.

I dug up some pictures of me as a toddler and a little kid, eyes sparkling with the kind of mischief only a toddler can get into, and I started thinking of my body as that little kid. I was responsible for *her*. I needed to take care of her—especially when she made bone-headed decisions like cancer. I could be mad and disappointed, yes, but look at that adorable, innocent face. She didn't know what she was doing.

Thinking about my body as a child I needed to take care of also helped me when it came to overwhelming emotions. When the fear or the anger threatened to take over my life, I looked at it like my toddler body was having a tantrum or being scared from a bad dream. The logical, rational, adult part of my brain could observe this, see it happening, and acknowledge it, but then also remember *it* was the adult. *It* was the part of me making the decisions, putting up the guardrails. My brain thought logically; my body didn't think at all.

After I realized that my body was just a toddler that I needed to take care of, this made it easier to forgive my body. Both for the cancer and the emotional outbursts. She hadn't done it *on purpose*. She didn't *mean* to kill us. She wasn't secretly out to get me. She was just a toddler, an Id, doing whatever felt right at the time.

Thinking this way helped me find some grace for myself. And grace is so important right now. Finding grace for yourself will help you find it for everyone else in your life: your spouse, your partner, your coworkers, your kids, your family, your caregivers, and healthcare providers. Everyone.

And in this tough time, everyone deserves a little grace.

When you start showing up for yourself—for your inner toddler—you will feel less betrayed.

Did you know the more you hate on yourself the worse you feel? Sounds logical, but most of us forget this. We hate on ourselves every day, second guess all our decisions, and stream a super critical line of thought in our heads all the time.

I know I've been so mean to myself in the past. I'm mean all the time—jeering at my failed attempts at writing, rolling my eyes at my less-than-stellar parenting moments, sighing about the people I dated when I was single, who did not deserve my affection or trust. I'm the first one to jump on the hate-on-me bandwagon.

I won't defend myself, but I'll defend my friends. I'm the first to jump in when my friends are too hard on themselves. I'll tell them to cut it out.

Treat yourself like you'd treat a friend. If your friend were angry at her body, furious even, wouldn't you step in and comfort her—tell her it's not her fault—or her body's fault? Give the same advice to yourself that you would give to your friend, sister, or neighbor.

And then start showing up for yourself. When you take care of your inner child, you'll start feeling better. Because if you don't take care of yourself, who will? If you are mean to yourself, who will be kind? This is where self-care comes in.

And you're already doing it. You're going to the medical appointments. That's self-care. You're reading this book, trying to get a handle on all the emotions. That's self-care. Keep on doing it. Keep on showing up. You will find that you'll feel better. You'll feel kinder to yourself. Because your body—the toddler—is throwing a tantrum. And most toddlers, when they throw a tantrum, feel out of control. They're testing the limits. Good parents put up guardrails so the toddler knows they are there, that they are loved and will be taken care of.

The more you set guardrails for your body, the more you show up and care for your body, the calmer you'll feel.

Pep talk #9:

Hey, Fighter. Have you been fighting yourself more than cancer lately? I get it. Mad at your body? Furious at the betrayal? We all feel this way. Be mad and then show yourself some grace. You (and your body) deserve it. You're fighting to live.

And, look, a house divided against itself can't stand. Cancer ISN'T your body, and it certainly isn't you. The enemy is cancer, not your body.

Shift your anger from your body to cancer. SHE's the real bitch. Hate on her all you want. Show up for your body because she deserves the care, and the more you do, the better you'll feel. I promise.

You are worth the fight. You are worth every ounce of energy. You are amazingly imperfect and worth fighting for.

Chapter Ten

The Only Way Is Through

"Cancer is the be-all and end-all of the sport, and the only thing you can do is show up to the game with your jersey on."

—Colleen Hoover

In this battle, you're going to get to a point where you feel like you can't go any further. Surgery, chemo, radiation. At some point, you'll feel like giving up. You'll be tired, pushed to the limit, and you'll feel like sitting down right there and not getting back up again.

Every single badass in this club had times when they thought they couldn't go on.

I cried in the shower so often I barely needed to turn the water on. I bargained SO damn hard—with myself, my doctors, the God I wasn't even sure was listening, with anyone and everyone. I clung to the idea that I could get out of this somehow.

Yet, I never found a shortcut.

I felt hopeless a million times. I felt I couldn't do what was asked of me. I believed the trial of my life had come, and I'd failed it.

The thing to remember is that, in this war against cancer, there will be skirmishes and battles that you'll lose. You won't be a gazelle leaping gracefully across the battlefield, avoiding every bullet and munition.

You'll get wounded.

You'll lose some battles—with yourself and with cancer.

But keep on fighting so you can win the war.

And to do that, you've got to keep moving.

With breast cancer, there's no way but through. The treatment will take as long as it takes. That's the hard truth. There are no shortcuts. Believe me, I looked for them all.

Still, I spent a lot of time at the beginning of my diagnosis bargaining with myself, with the universe, with my doctors.

Maybe I *don't* need the chemo; maybe I don't have to do the double mastectomy; maybe I could try some herbal tea instead... If I only just ate better, exercised, and just did juice cleanses for the rest of my life, then I won't have to do any painful treatments, right? I promised God and the universe I'd be a better person. I would. Just give me the easy way out.

I spent a lot of time trying to wish away what was happening to me, but it never worked. But here's a little secret—once you're done with the bargaining and trying to find an escape hatch, and you get to acceptance... THEN you can really get to the hard work of fighting this bitch.

I feel like I'm losing my mind.
"I'm just all over the place," I tell my counselor in our session. "I'm angry. I'm sad. I'm terrified. I'm like a ping-pong ball of emotions." One day, I'm so angry. The next day, sad. "I also realize that I've been trying to make some kind of deal with myself. Like the surgery will be fine because I'll get perkier, better boobs. But it's not okay. None of this is okay. It's not a good trade."

"You're feeling a lot of different things," she notes.

"All the things. I'm feeling all the things."

"Cara." She pauses and looks at me, head slightly cocked. "You're grieving. I'm sure if you look at all the stages, you'll see. You're grieving."

She's so right. It becomes so clear.

Denial. Anger. Bargaining. Depression. Acceptance.

They're all there. To varying degrees.

"You're grieving. The death hasn't happened yet, but you know it's coming. Your loved ones are on life support, and you're grieving ahead of time. This is what you're doing. You're moving through all the stages, and they don't always happen in order."

She's right.

She's so right.

There's something in me that breaks open then. The sobs come, and it all makes sense. I am grieving. I'm grieving the loss of trust in my body. I'm grieving the loss of my breasts. I'm grieving all they've meant to me. I'm grieving the loss of whatever I had before, the life I had pre-cancer. I'm grieving my healthy self. I'm grieving the loss of feeling immortal. I'm grieving it all.

Mood swings will give you whiplash.

One minute, you'll be fine, the next, furious, and the next, sad and defeated.

You're grieving the loss of your breasts (or part of them). You're grieving the loss of your pre-cancer self (the one whose problems seem so small and inconsequential now). You're grieving the loss of your health (Oh, did you take it for granted back then!). You're grieving the loss of trust with your body (remember Chapter Nine). You're grieving.

That means you'll at some point or another go through all the stages of grief:

- **Denial**—I don't have cancer. You have cancer. There must be some mistake. Cancer doesn't run in my family. I don't even have the gene! Could the tests be wrong? I didn't like the way the radiologist handled that biopsy. Where did he get his degree again? Surely, there has to be some mistake. Also, maybe if I just ignore it, it'll go away? Hello, sand, meet head!

- **Anger**—Cancer? What the holy hell? Fuck Cancer. Fuck Everyone. Why Me? Fuck everyone and everything, especially the scheduling nurse. Why can't she get me in sooner? And my partner can't even unload the damn dishwasher?! I have fucking cancer?! The fuck?! Cancer sucks. *I want Cancer dead. I want its family dead. I want to burn its house to the ground. I want to go over in the middle of the night and piss on its ashes!* (Courtesy of Al Capone in *The Untouchables*.)

- **Bargaining**—Okay. Maybe if I just change my diet, the cancer will go away. How about this? I promise to eat right, cut out alcohol (seriously this time, not just for dry January when I cheated anyway), and I'll go to every doctor's appointment I ever skipped before. Hey, what if I go to church? Will that help me? I'll do anything.

- **Depression**—I can't bargain my way out of this. Shit. I've really got Big C Cancer. I'm fucked. Everything is awful. I'm probably going to die. And even if I live, what kind of life will I have without boobs? I don't want to get out of bed. I don't want to do anything. What's the point? I'm dying. Everything is horrible forever. Nothing will ever be cured. My life is over.

- **Acceptance**—Well, I've tried to deny, bargain, rage, and wallow my way to a different answer, but I still have cancer. It's not going away, so I guess I'd better kick cancer's ass.

One of the biggest obstacles you'll face is your own morale.
Cancer will find ways to disappoint you even when you KNOW it's disappointing.

There's so much fucking disappointment with cancer. It's the truth. You think that you can't be more disappointed than getting the news you've got cancer, but trust me, you can. The cancer diagnosis can get worse. The treatment can feel medieval. The small ray of hope and light you clung to disappears and you're sinking down into the darkness again.

Because this is CANCER. It fucking sucks. There are a million ways cancer can continue to disappoint you.

With the lymph node biopsy.

The size of the tumor when they cut it out of you.

Your upset stomach from chemo during that important Zoom call.

Your hair growing back weirdly curly.

Your fingernails peeling straight off from chemo.

The skin infection ON YOUR FACE from immunotherapy.

Ah, the list goes on and on.

It's hard to keep a positive attitude. And you know what? You don't have to be a ray of sunshine.

You just have to be a bad motherfucker who is going to stubbornly push her way through. Be bossy as hell. Be aggressive all you want. Be NOT nice in a way that your aunt would disapprove of.

There's no way but through.

Make a Plan for Yourself When Your Treatment Is Done

To get to the other side, to make it through, it helps to dangle a carrot for yourself.

Let me tell you a story about Taylor Swift and the Eras Tour.

My youngest daughter counts herself among the most dedicated Swifties there ever was or ever will be. She knows every lyric to every single song and has been listening to Tay Tay since she'd been a toddler. I was a fan, but she was a

MEGA fan. My husband and I sat online, waiting to get tickets for her Soldier Field performance in Chicago, but after hours of trying, we failed to secure tickets. Resellers asked for $2,500 or more a seat ($1,000 if you wanted a completely obstructed view), and this mom just couldn't do that. And then the concert came and went, and we saw hundreds of photos of her friends having the time of their lives. My daughter was so sad, but she said, "Don't worry, Mom. It's okay."

And my teen began to learn to drive, insisting Taylor Swift (Taylor's version, what else?) be exclusively played in the car "because it helped her concentrate." *Midnights* became the background of taking slow turns in empty parking lots. Taylor was again the soundtrack of our lives. Then came the announcement of the European leg of the Eras Tour. Lo and behold, there was a stop in London, just days after her school trip to Europe ended, and I could get tickets. We could extend their trip, take a train to London. . . yet, I hesitated. Should I? The airfare and hotel. . .

My husband said, "This is the tour of a lifetime. Do it."

You never regret an amazing memory.

And so we got tickets in the nosebleeds, third from the top, but IN THE STADIUM, and I held on to them for months because it was going to be said daughter's Christmas present. *Surprise! You're going to see Taylor Swift after all. . . IN LONDON.*

This was a pack-it-on-the-credit-cards, hope-to-pay-for-it-later situation.

And that might be the end of the story right there. But then came a routine mammogram when doctors told me. . . I had cancer.

And I didn't know if I'd be well enough to go.

It felt like I'd let her down. Like I'd somehow let the whole family down. That's what cancer feels like. Cancer is scary and awful, and it tests you in ways you never thought you'd ever be tested. But what it does, more than anything, is help you get crystal clear about what's important in your life. It helps you see what's noise and what isn't. And what I knew was that I would kick cancer. For my husband. For my family. For my children.

And for Taylor Swift, dammit.

I was going to drag myself there, come hell or high water.

The concert would be five months after the double mastectomy and three months after chemo. I'd be in the middle of immunotherapy, but. . . it could be done.

So, I got the double mastectomy. I went through the chemo. And the immunotherapy. I did everything I could possibly do, and at each stage, I told my doctors: "I have to be well come the end of June. I HAVE to be okay. I have to take my daughter to see Taylor Swift in London."

It might sound silly, but it wasn't. The concert became the thing I could focus on during the bad days. The nauseous days. The tired days. The foggy days. The painful days. I had to be well. I was GOING to be well. I was taking my daughter to Wembley to see Taylor Swift, dammit. I was DOING THIS.

And you know what? The doctors and nurses all GOT IT. They got right on board. They were Swifties themselves, or they had their own Swifties at home. Or, even more importantly, they knew the importance of a patient with a plan, with a goal, determined to be well. They understood the stakes immediately, and they worked out a plan to help me get there.

And the treatment wasn't easy, but it was hard to feel sorry for myself when I had the world's most popular show to attend.

On the worst days, I knew there were brighter ones ahead. I knew on the other end of awful, my daughter would get to see her idol. I was going to see my daughter scream-sing every damn lyric to every damn song at Wembley. Hell, I was going to scream-sing them myself!

And I did it. I beat cancer, just in time, and we went. And it was a dream. When those first few notes of "Miss Americana & the Heartbreak Prince" rang out over the heads of the 85,000+ sold-out crowd at Wembley, she sang, "It's been a long time coming. . ."

Oh boy, sister. If you only knew just how long.

Tears stung my eyes. The road here had been long and painful. But the moment was. . . finally here. And the show was amazing. Taylor Swift did not disappoint. And my daughter knew every word to every song. She sang herself hoarse. She glowed. She levitated. It was a memory I know she'll carry with her for all time. That I will, too. It was everything and more.

So, you may not have an Eras Tour performance to look forward to.

But you can make some plans. Later on down the road. Have a bright goal to look forward to—for you or someone near and dear to you.

The Other Side

Whether or not you have a fantastic concert or trip planned for the other side, it's important to believe you WILL get to the other side.

Back to your old life, your imperfect, stressful, amazing life. When your kids and husband aren't worried about you. Where your friends aren't whispering, "How is she *really* doing?"

And then you can make plans. You can make ALL the fucking plans, not worried that there will be a biopsy/treatment/surgery needed and have to cancel. Not crossing my fingers and HOPING I can make that concert/book signing/vacation.

I'd like to make fucking plans.

I'd like to not worry 24/7.

I want my old life back. The one where I didn't, more than occasionally, think about mortality.

I want that life back.

That's the other side.

The treatments will feel like they last forever, but for many of you, they'll be a year or eighteen months.

That's a blink when it comes to the timeline of your life. Would you give a year or eighteen months of hell so you can have twenty or thirty healthy years?

Of course, you would.

Now, others of you will be on treatment for the rest of your life. I know this because at the chemo center, we didn't ring a loud bell. I got a tiny bell that I rang outside the door of the center because some people inside would never get to ring the bell.

That's just the fact of the matter.

But they will get to live—a helluva lot longer than they would've thirty years ago, when breast cancer was pretty much a death sentence.

But for the rest of you, whose treatment is temporary, keep in mind you're putting in the hard work for a few months or a year so that you can get your life back. And, yes, none of our lives will be the same. We'll be on a cancer watch for the rest of it. None of us truly get beyond cancer. It's always there, a threat, lying in wait.

But the hard work of battling cancer is now.

I diligently crossed off twelve chemotherapy treatments on the calendar, and then twenty-six immunotherapy treatments, as well as two biopsies, one port insertion, a double mastectomy, and a reconstruction surgery, all over the course of fifteen months. In those fifteen months, I felt the treatment would never end.

And then. . . it did.

And I'll tell you, it was like waking up from a fever dream, not even sure it was all real.

"Was that it? Really? I'm all done?"

For those whom the treatment continues...

For those of you on treatment for the rest of your life—I salute you. I salute your damn tenacity, and your willingness to do what it takes to survive. You're a bad ass. Period. This fight never ends for you.

I see you.

Your new normal is a forever normal.

I hope you're holding on to your joy, your verve for life, and that the side effects are minimal. That you've made peace with it all. I hope you've found new joys in new places, and most of all, I'm so glad you're still here. With us. At the infusion center and everywhere else.

Odds are made to be beaten.

For those of you in later stages of cancer, being told your odds aren't good, I challenge you to look back on a time in your life when you did beat the odds. When you got the A, got into that college, got that promotion, landed that job, went on that date, avoided that car accident, won at that Las Vegas craps table— whatever it was, you've beaten the odds before.

You can do it again.

Odds are just odds. They don't dictate the course of your life. They're just numbers. That's all. They're not your fate. They're not you.

There's no way but through.

You can be scared. Of the pain. Of all the things that can go wrong.

But we still have to go.

You can be angry. Why me? Why is this happening? I don't deserve this.

But we still have to go.

You can be sad, so sad. I don't want to cut off parts of me. I don't want to lose the parts that make me, me.

But we still have to go.

You can be petulant. You don't wanna go. You didn't ask for this. You don't want it. I know.

But we still have to go.

You can be worried. Anxious. Panicky. What's going to be next? When is the next shoe going to drop? When do I hear more bad news?

But we still have to go.

You can be scared. Terrified. What if none of this works? What if it all goes wrong?

But, self, we still have to go.

We have to go because there is no choice.

We can't stay here. We can't sit down. We've got to keep moving.

There's no way but through.

There's no way, but straight through.

We can go, scared and screaming.

We can go, angry and yelling.

We can go, sad and crying.

We can go, petulant and pouting.

We can go, worried and anxious.

We can go, terrified and howling.

But we've got to go.

We can go feeling all these things, but we've got to go. We've got to go straight through.

If we stay, if we sit down, we die.

So, we've got to go.

Pep talk #10:

Hey, Battle-tested Badass. Is the battle wearing you down? Are you so damn tired and desperate for an off ramp? I looked for one every single day of sixteen months of treatment.

The only way is through. You've got to walk through the fire. There's no other way.

The good news is you won't be in the fire forever. You won't be in hell forever. Keep putting one foot in front of the other and you will eventually walk yourself straight out of this hellscape and into your amazing life on the other side.

The key is to keep moving.

One step at a time.

You'll get there.

Chapter Eleven
Bye-Bye Boobs. It's Been Real.

"Never be ashamed of a scar. It simply means you were stronger than whatever tried to hurt you."

—Unknown

So, this is the chapter about my double mastectomy. If you aren't ready for this, or if mastectomy is NOT on the menu for you, then—skip right on ahead. I won't be mad.

If you're just not ready to even think about mastectomy yet, even if your doctor recommends it, that's okay, too. Skip on to the next chapter.

Many of you will be able to do a lumpectomy and be fine. My cancer was too spread out in the left breast for that, and the intraductal tumor was too big, at two inches long. My husband took one look at my mammogram and said, "That looks like a starry sky." And it did. My surgeon recommended a mastectomy for the left.

And then I had to decide—do I keep the other one?

This is a deeply personal decision, and there is no right answer for all.

I know of women who opted to do a lumpectomy instead of doctor's orders for a mastectomy because they simply didn't want to say goodbye to their breasts.

I get it.

The thing is—I won't judge anybody's decisions. They're YOUR personal decision. You don't want to cut your boobs off? They're YOUR boobs. You get to decide! You'd rather die than go under the knife? YOUR life. You get to decide.

I cannot stress this enough.

I decided for the double mastectomy because I wanted to live. I have a blended family of five children. Three of whom were still in high school. And then there was my beautiful, amazing husband, PJ, who pleaded with me not to leave him alone with the loud, boisterous, chaotic circus that is our family. "This is a house of cards that will fall without you," he said.

I wasn't ready to dip and leave them all stranded.

My mom said I'd feel differently if I was in my seventies, like she was. Maybe I wouldn't fight so hard. Or maybe I would. I don't know.

So, what I'm trying to tell you is that it's your life, your decision.

I had to have a mastectomy, but I opted for a double— because there was frankly no way I was going to sit through another suspicious mammogram or biopsy ever again. Something in me said, "No, fucking way. Not ever."

That was my True No (*Defy* by Dr. Sunita Sah).

One boob had already gone awol, and there was no fucking way I was trusting the second to behave. Also, while I realize some women opt to get partial reconstruction (have one fake boob and one real) I just didn't believe this would work out well for me. I wanted to be back to normal as soon as I could. I was fifty, and that meant that I felt I still had some beach years ahead of me. I wanted reconstruction.

But again, that's my choice.

For those women who opt not to get reconstruction— that's 100% fine, too.

But as you make that decision, ensure that you're doing so clear-eyed and not muddled by fear.

For some women, breasts are essential to their identity.

I'd always been a b-cup, and that meant that I never had extra boobage, the kind that spilled over in push-up bras, or cleavage for miles, and I'd always lamented that they weren't as big as they could be. I always had gaps between me and the cups; I never fully filled anything. I envied my D or DD or FF friends, with their hourglass figures that burst straight out of button-up shirts. I never had a problem wearing button-up shirts.

To be honest with you, I hated my boobs. They arrived late to the party, never grew to their full potential, and had the audacity to stay cone-shaped instead of the preferred perky and round. People my size—hovering between an A and B cup, desperate for ALL the padding—sometimes thought about augmentation. But I hated the idea of surgery. Someone cutting on me while I slept? NO, thank you. Plus, my mom—who hates doctors—(have I mentioned that?)—always liked to point out that surgery wasn't just for fun. My dad, the surgeon, also said the same thing. Sometimes people didn't wake up from the anesthetic. Save the surgery for when you really need it.

So, I did.

I eventually had two daughters and, during that time, found out that my smaller than average titties actually were amazing milk producers. Some women had trouble with that, but I didn't. And then, I thought—*Hey, girls, let's have a truce.* I hated on you—wrongly—because you did an amazing job at feeding my babies, which despite what PornHub wants to tell you, is actually their purpose. So, thank you.

And then, cancer.

These bitches are trying to kill me! What the fuck?!

I thought we had a truce, ladies. I thought we *agreed*. But my girls held a grudge, I guess from my teen years when I hated on them, stuffing tissues between them.

Who am I without breasts?

"I'm worried I'll not just lose my breasts," I tell my counselor. "I worry I'll lose myself. I'll become a different person. A bitter person, or a sad person, or just lose my joy. I'll lose my. . ."

"Soul?"

I nod.

"When I was in graduate school, there was a professor—I hated this professor—he told us: tell me where the soul is. Is it in the brain? Show me. Where? Is it in the heart? Where? Show me. And of course, no one could show him."

She rolls her eyes, indicating he was a pompous, know-it-all, but he was also right.

"But the point is, your soul isn't on the table. Your soul is *yours*. It can't be taken from you. Surgeons can't cut it out. It's yours."

As smooth as a Barbie Doll.

"We might not be able to save the nipples," my surgeon said in a pre-op visit. "But we're going to try."

I never thought about not having nipples, about having boobs as smooth as Barbie.

"You can get nipple reconstruction. Or nipple tattoos," she said.

Nipple tattoos?

I don't want to be here anymore.

"I'll be smooth as a Barbie," I complain to my husband, PJ.

He just grins. "Well, I'm pretty much as smooth as a Ken doll down there, so we'll be perfect match."

Your scars will be your badges of heroism.

This sounds like a load of shit.

But it's true.

Your scars are your badges of courage.

I didn't want to look at mine, I'll be honest with you. After surgery, I looked down the first time, shivered in revulsion, and then immediately looked away. If I had been forced to stare at my scars all day long in the mirror, I would've gone mad. It was a mangled, scarred mess, with black stitching. Flat and horrible and awful. I WAS living with a horror movie, just without all the unsettling music.

"It's okay," the nurse told me. "You don't have to look. You don't ever have to look."

And you know what? I really didn't look after that. My husband helped me clean my scars. He's a fucking hero. I apologized to him so often, but he said, "This is just temporary," and he was right. This wouldn't be what I looked like forever.

And even now, after the reconstruction, I still have scars. But now when I see them, they don't scare me. They don't repulse me. They've healed and faded a little, but when I look at them, they show me that I'm tough.

That I faced some hard fucking decisions and didn't flinch (or flinch that often).

That the cancer tried to kill me, but I survived.

You can lose your boobs without losing yourself.

I know you know this, but your boobs are not actually who you are.

They're not even what make you a woman.

And what makes you a woman? Is it your uterus? Your ovaries? Your vagina or your clit? Your clothes or your makeup? Is it because you simply feel like a woman on the inside? There are a million ways you can define being a woman that don't have anything to do with your breasts.

Your boobs are one piece of you, but they're not *you*, the essential *you*, your soul, that energy signature that lives on forever in the universe, the irreplaceable you.

That part of you, the surgeon can never touch.

Neither can the cancer.

That part of you is *always* you and cannot be cut away.

Make a list of the things that make you, *you*. Are you crafty? A planner? Do you love to cook? Do you like to organize things? Are you the life of the party in your group? Are you funny? Are you serious? Do you like to read? Are you an introvert? An extrovert? Do you love to travel? Are you a homebody? Can you mix a mean cocktail? Do you shred the guitar? Do you make pottery? Do you garden? Do you live to tour haunted houses? Are you stubborn? Easy going? What are the hobbies and traits that make you, *you*?

None of those things involve boobs.

You can even love to flirt—and not have boobs.

You're not losing *you*; you're simply losing a part of your body. A part that, thankfully, you don't need to survive (like your brain, heart, lungs, or liver).

The thing is surgery and losing your boobs can feel like a horror movie. It's awful and terrible, but there's also something good there.

Imagine if you had cancer in your brain or your stomach or your lungs?

You don't need your breasts to think.

Or eat.

Or breathe.

Or hear.

Or sing.

Or see.

You don't need them to run. Or kayak. Or swim. Or lay by the pool and order margaritas.

They're nice accessories, don't get me wrong, and maybe they're your very favorite accessories.

But they're just that. They're not essential. It doesn't mean we don't love them and we won't miss them, but it means we'll be able to do so much without them. If leaving them behind means you have many more years—or decades even—of running and laughing and hugging and sharing and traveling and living, then isn't that time—that precious time—worth the sacrifice?

Your spouse should love you with or without boobs.
Would you love your spouse if they suddenly lost a leg? Of course, you would. Because you love the person, not just the person's body. When you gaze lovingly into your spouse's eyes, you're not thinking about a specific body part (usually).

"I don't care whether you have boobs or not; I care that you LIVE," PJ said many times.

How bad is it?
I know some of you want the full, unvarnished truth about the double-mastectomy. How fucking bad is it? It's not great. But you can do it. You can. Here's the rundown.

They will try to rush you the fuck out of the hospital.
Gone are the days that you can choke down hospital food for three days while someone gives you the good drugs through the IV for forty-eight hours. A double mastectomy is considered a day surgery. Outpatient.

That's right.

You read that right.

They want you in and out same day.

I am NOT a doctor, but I think they want you out because studies show the longer you stay in the hospital the worse your recovery rate is. They want you AWAY from the antibiotic-resistant killer bacteria that festers in hospitals and back home walking around, getting better sleep than you will attached to a damn beeping machine.

When it comes to having someone with you at the hospital to drive you home MAKE SURE it's the person who will be helping you with your FUCKING drains (sorry, I can't mention drains and not curse. You'll know what I mean when you get them.).

You'll be loopy on post-operative meds (or super nauseous because—anesthetic) when the nurses try to explain how you will care for these motherfuckers, and you'll need a sober person with attention to detail. Get your spouse AND your sister in there. Get your best friend. Whomever will be ON IT.

If you are terrified to go home with these open wounds and drains an hour after the operating room table, ask to stay.
This is an option. Some people want to get out of the hospital as fast as fucking possible, and other people want some nurse care before they do.

In my situation, the surgery before me went hours over, so the plastic surgeon asked me if I wanted to go ahead and stay overnight, since I'd be headed home at like 11 p.m. I opted to stay overnight.

The sleep sucked, and—like all hospital stays—attendants woke me every hour or so to check my vitals or drain the drains. I had one very cranky overnight nurse who seemed to empty the drains with extra hard tugs like *I* was her asshole boss. I mean, I didn't assign you this shift, ma'am. I know you hate your life, but. . . what did I do to you?

I got crappy sleep, but I was also glad to be there, to get multiple close-up examples of how to drain the drains.

Anesthetic also makes me nauseous AF, so having IV meds to combat that was good.

If you want to stay at the hospital, ask your doctor if it's an option.

The nurses all told me to walk—they were right.

Before they let me leave the hospital, the nurse asked me to take a slow, shuffling walk up and down the corridor of the hospital.

"The more you move, the faster you'll heal," she told me as I walked slowly up and down the tiled hallway.

She was right.

When I got home, I made a point of getting up regularly from bed and walking in circles inside for five or ten minutes at a time, gradually working up to when I could do fifteen. I made little slow shuffling circles around our kitchen and attached dining room. This wasn't running a 5K, but it was getting the blood moving and helping me heal.

And I did as much as I was able, pain permitting, and I felt it did help. It also helps reduce your risk of lymphedema, a common side effect of losing lymph nodes. That's when you get swelling in your extremities, and it's not great, so doing what we can to avoid that is a good idea.

The pain from the mastectomy wasn't as bad as I feared.

This is not true for everyone, but it was true for me. The pain (of the actual surgical scars and the breasts) was bad, but not AS bad as I worried about. This was mainly because they scraped out every single nerve-ending. They saved my nipples, but I cannot feel them. Not one bit. You could light one on fire and I wouldn't know. I do not feel the skin, either. The nurses told me that I'd need to be careful about cuts or scrapes or burns. That I wouldn't be able to feel anything in case I'd gotten a bug bite or a scrape, and I'd need to be extra vigilant so that nothing was infected.

The pain was deeper (below the surface) like a bruise against my inner chest wall, where the expanders (the placeholders for part one of reconstruction, which make a pocket in the chest, and are also slowly expanded over time with regular shots of saline solution), were sewn into my chest. These things were about as comfortable as wearing champagne coasters under your skin. I felt them every single day, and it was—as one nurse said—an iron bra you can never take off.

I was supposed to only wear them for a month to six weeks and then have reconstruction surgery, but—Surprise! I needed chemo!—so I'd have to wait nine months with them in. Not fun. Zero stars. Do NOT recommend.

All that said, the pain—generally—wasn't sharp. It was dull and always there, thudding in the background, creeping up on me all day until early evening when I just wanted to be under the covers in bed.

Because of this, I actually never took the heavy-duty pain-killers. I didn't want to be constipated on top of being uncomfortable, and I also didn't want to get hooked on oxy. It's unlikely you'll get enough to get hooked on, but it is likely they'll make you constipated AF. And, well, I just didn't need something else on top of everything. I popped a lot of Tylenol instead.

The annoying, never-ending, wincing little pricks from the FUCKING drains, however, is like water torture.

If you have a double mastectomy, you'll likely have four FUCKING drains—two on each side. Think plastic tubing attached to a little clear rubber ball (like the worst bloodiest stress ball on earth). Apparently, when you cut off a big part of your body, your body's like, *What the fuck? Let me fill it with. . . blood-tinged fluid!* So, the drains are there to help your body get used to the fact you don't have boobs anymore. The drains FUCKING SUCK. I am not going to lie to you. They are the worst.

Also, they feel medieval. Like, we haven't come up with a better way to do this than a tube stitched to an open wound. WTF?! We've got the entire history of humankind in a little device in our palms, but we're still using the technique invented in *400 BC* by the Greek doctor Hippocrates.—Yeah, you know, the one who wrote that do-no-harm oath?![38]

The FUCKING drains are the worse because it's a small little incision, but it's open, and I felt a constant little prick of pain every time I moved (or sometimes even just breathed), and by the end of the day, I was exhausted, frustrated, and ready to pull the damn tubes out myself. Don't do this by the way. The doctor WILL know.

You also have to empty these FUCKING drains every few hours.

They suck. I hate them. FUCKING drains. They got caught on my shirt; the tube tangled against the skin on my stomach or tugged when stuck in the waistband of my flannel PJ bottoms. I fucking DROPPED one, once, and it hung FROM MY SKIN, swinging by my knees like I was a grandfather clock from hell.

Getting two drains out.

"Some people tell me that they fell out." The physician's assistant rolls her eyes. I'm at my follow-up appointment at the plastic surgeon's office, and I'm looking at the tube she pulled out of me—at least eight inches long? No, that shit doesn't just fall out. It's maybe stomped or tugged out, but it doesn't "fall."

---

[38] "A History of Thoracic Drainage: From Ancient Greeks to Wound Sucking Drummers to Digital Monitoring," Sarah Walcott-Sapp, CTS Net, April 9, 2015.

But I understand why some women, frustrated, rip them out in a fit of rage. It took every ounce of patience I had not to. Because I wanted to heal, and I certainly didn't want an infection. Plus, I didn't want to prolong this hell any more than I had to. Every day sucks, but then you're closer to getting a pair out, and then the other pair. Then you'll have this tiny little scabs, and you'll wonder what all the fuss was about.

For those of you who haven't yet had surgery and are still with me, don't freak out.

Feel the need to freak out? Channel the freak-out into prep.

So, there are a million things you can do or buy to prepare yourself for a double or single mastectomy. Let's start with a shopping list—not the fun kind, but still. Here are some of the things I found the MOST helpful, ranked from MOST helpful to least:

1. **A heated bidet toilet seat.** The kind with a remote that shoots warm water *back there* to help get you clean. Look, we're friends now, surely, so I can share private details like this with you. Your range of motion will be limited right after surgery. And I didn't really feel like asking for my husband's help down there, okay? Some things need to remain a mystery—until I'm ninety years old and incontinent.

2. **Zip up/button up the front shirts.** I opted for special ones with little interior pockets to hold the FUCKING drains. Giving them their own pocket to live in helps. You can sew your own pocket into a zip-up fleece you don't care to keep or you can find fancy ones online that are likely way overpriced. But you can also grab some old flannel button-ups from your partner's closet or the thrift store.

3. **Special pillows.** There are so many of these online, but I found sleep and seatbelt ones the most helpful. You can probably also use some throw pillows you already have around the house if you don't want to buy new ones. Also, a throw pillow or even a folded jacket between you and the seatbelt also works. That seatbelt hurt me for the first few weeks after surgery, but they might not hurt you. Pillows came in handy, too, when I needed something to help me sleep. Mostly to keep myself stationary because any movement activated the twinge of those FUCKING drains. I found propping myself up on my back was the best way to keep me from waking up in the middle of the night.

4. **Extra lanyards.** The drains can hook onto a simple lanyard (any one from any convention you ever went to can do), so that the lanyard takes the weight of the drains and not your incision. The whole point is to make sure the tubes aren't tugging on your skin. Interior pockets also help carry the weight of the bulbs. Some people will find the interior pockets more comfortable than the lanyards, but you WILL need a lanyard for the shower.

5. **Super comfy—anything.** Maybe grab yourself some amazing (front zip/button up) pajamas, or extra fuzzy socks (with tread – you might be unsteady!).

Going under the knife.

"God, that was a terrible case," complained my breast surgeon when she rushed into my pre-op stall at the hospital, three hours past the time I was supposed to go in. My breast surgeon was flustered. She'd run into complications during the double mastectomy before mine, and she was HOURS late. I'd been sitting in my pre-op horse stall with the curtain in my hospital-issued gown and bright yellow socks with the tread to reduce slippage for *hours*. "I hope yours is easier," she grumbles.

Uh. . . me, too?

My surgeon looked exhausted, beat, after a two-hour surgery took seven hours, and now she had to cut into me?

Eek.

My dad, the orthopedic surgeon, had already told me that good surgeons turn something on when they're tired and exhausted, something the rest of us don't usually have. A fifth gear. Dad said, when he had a marathon surgical case, he was *extra* careful when he was tired because he knew he was tired. He had to be *extra* vigilant so that's usually when he did his best surgeries.

Or he was just telling me this on the phone, so I didn't panic when I was wheeled in the OR.

One final thing before surgery—write a letter to your boobs.
I know this sounds ridiculous. But it does help. Say an official goodbye to your boobs. You can write them a letter, or talk to them in the mirror, whatever it is that feels right to you. Say your official goodbye. Here's the letter I wrote to mine:

Goodbye, Boobs.
Hey there, Boobs. Breasts. Titties. Bosoms.

Whatever your preferred name.

We don't talk that often. Although, lately, we've been talking a lot. Especially you, Lefty.

Look, I know we haven't always had a great relationship. I mean, when I was ten, all I did was dream about your arrival. What would you be? Big? Bigger? Perky? Would you have personality? Would you defy gravity? Or need extra firm support?

165

You would, without a doubt, make me a Woman. Sure, everyone else filled me with lies about periods making you a Woman, but everyone knew that, when you arrived, I'd wear a bra, and then I'd officially be a Woman because that's when people on the *outside* could see I wasn't a girl anymore. I'd had a period since I was ten, and everyone still thought I was a pip squeak kid.

All of my friends got theirs before I got mine. Exaggeration? I think not. I was fourteen before you arrived, and I had friends on their third or fourth generation of bras by then.

There was all that dramatic build-up, but let's face it: you were a disappointment, Boobs.

A-cup at best. Cleavage was impossible without a sick amount of duct tape and, even then, barely any. I tried to trot you out.

I was cis-straight, and I soon found out that whatever small morsels you were offering were really only acceptable to Ass Men. Boob Men were not interested in you. It's a sad fact, but true. Ass Men didn't really care, ergo, their names.

I strapped you (easily) into sports bras and took you through 10K races. I stuffed you into push-up bras. I fretted about how you looked in a bikini.

Then, I got pregnant for the first time. Now, suddenly, you grew. And grew.

You transformed. You'd failed me before, no doubt, but I discovered something magical about you. You weren't show-ers Or growers. You were Doers. You made milk. So much milk. Milk that flowed so much that my baby gained so much weight the doctors were impressed. I never had to worry about you not doing your job.

I realized I'd underestimated you. I'd misunderstood you. You were amazing. You fed two babies for their first year of life. That's a lot of milk.

Sure, my nipples bled. Sure, I got a clogged duct now and again, but you kept on fighting. Kept on feeding. You were miraculous.

And then, I thought, we had a truce. I was never going to cut you open and stuff implants in you because you'd nourished our babies. You might not be the biggest or best or perkiest, but you were mine.

Then came the mammograms. I know you didn't like them. The techs didn't either as they squished you into a position on a plastic press that just wasn't designed to accommodate you.

I found out you were dense then. You gave me numerous scares over the years. I always needed two mammograms—one was never enough with you, drama queen.

Then, they found the cancer.

I get that you wanted to live forever. That's what cancer is, after all, cells that refuse to die. Boobs, you wanted immortality.

But you can't have it.

Because you're killing me. I'm mad at you about that. I thought we had a deal.

But I also get it.

Still, I'm letting you go. I'm letting the doctors take you so I can live. I need boobs, yes, but I don't need *you*, in particular. I'm going to get new ones. I've got more living to do.

I want to thank you for all you've done. You fed my babies, made me feel like a woman for many years. Been a part of me.

Now, I'm going to release you.

Pep talk #11:

Hey, my Kick-ass Fighter. How you doing? Saying goodbye is always hard, and saying goodbye to something as essential as your boobs can seem impossible. Take all the time you need. This is hard. Nothing about it is easy.

But you've done hard things before.

Maybe harder than this, maybe not, but you've said hard goodbyes.

This goodbye has a definite silver lining. You're saying goodbye to your boob or boobs so you can say hello to the rest of your life. Your boobs are making the ultimate sacrifice so you can stay with us.

You are not your boobs. You are so much more.

Keep your eye on the prize. This is pain for gain. This is a goodbye to part of you so the rest of you can fucking live.

Chapter Twelve
Chemo—Time to Spin the Wheel of Misfortune

"Without hair, a queen is still a queen."

—Prajakta Mhadnak

"No hair, don't care."

—unknown

I was so relieved when my breast surgeon told me they'd got all the cancer—clean margins!—and it hadn't spread to my lymph node, that I let my guard down. Technically, I was cancer-free—there was no detectible cancer in my body as of that moment.

It was a moment to celebrate.

Until it wasn't.

"So what next?" I asked my breast surgeon. I was hoping she'd tell me to go home and celebrate. Do I get to ring a bell now? Wasn't I out of the woods?

Chemo had been a specter hovering over my life since diagnosis. I'd gone through a battery of tests where at each stage they really seemed to be pushing me to chemo (if the biopsy of the lymph node found cancer, then chemo first, then surgery, or if the ultrasound or MRI found a bigger tumor, then it we'd need to shrink it with chemo BEFORE surgery and on and on). I'd flown through those tests by the skin of my teeth, but I'd made it. I'd had surgery first. Not chemo.

Before surgery, my doctor had warned me: We could still find cancer in a lymph node. The tumor could still be big. We might need multiple surgeries, or I might still need chemo. Or radiation.

But then she told me the tumor wasn't bigger than they thought. And the lymph node was clean. She told me I didn't need radiation.

"Thank God," I said because my plastic surgeon had told me how radiation affects implants. The scar tissue means the implants might not sit right, if at all, ever. "And what about chemo? This means I don't need chemo, right?"

"You're a borderline case," my surgeon tried to warn me. "With the size of the tumor, it's a gray area. . ." She sucked in a breath. "You should just talk to your oncologist about it."

✧　✧　✧

After healing up, getting those FUCKING drains out, and going to physical therapy so that I could once more lift my arm higher than my shoulder, I was feeling pretty good. The expanders the plastic surgeon put into my chest as placeholders were annoying every single day (you try wearing an iron bra that felt as if it was a medieval torture device), but I was cancer-free. I was even heading to my plastic surgeon regularly to get the expanders filled, so my chest started to look... semi-normal again.

I'd been on the worst ride of my life for the last ten weeks, and I was just glad to give myself the hope that maybe, just maybe, all the hard stuff was behind me.

But then I went to visit the oncologist. I was fully expecting a rubber stamp. I don't know *why* I was expecting a rubber stamp. Nothing about the process so far was rubber-stamped anything. I'd been running worst-case scenarios in my brain at all hours of the day and night for three months, so I don't know why, at that moment, I choose to be blithely optimistic. I guess it was because I felt like they'd done the worst to me. They cut off my boobs. What's really all that terrible next to that?

Surely, that IS the worst.

I'm the first to admit that I went into that appointment totally overconfident.

I missed it by two millimeters.

My invasive tumors (the ones outside the milk ducts) were 5 mm and 2 mm. To put it in perspective for Americans because our weights and measures make no fucking sense, 5mm is less than a *quarter of an inch*.

The intraductal tumor happened to reach 49 mm (that was 1.9 inches). But they don't usually care how big that one is— all those bitches are at the original bar. They care about the bitches that sneak out to the street (the mass in the breast tissue surrounding the ducts).

The oncologist told me this:

If my invasive tumor had been 3 mm, then she would've patted me on the back and told me to go home. No chemo, no further treatment.

If the invasive tumor was 6 mm, then all the studies and research say the chance of recurrence is much higher, and I'd need chemotherapy, combined with immunotherapy. I'd need chemo, for sure. Look at the research.

But mine was 5mm.

"So, my reasoning is, you're closer to 6 than 3, so you should do the chemo."

I blinked fast. I glanced at my husband. Was it time to go into the white room? Maybe.

"But there are lots of kinds of chemo," I said because I'd actually read a little bit of information in the Worst Phonebook of All Time. In that I learned not every chemo is the lose your hair/fingernails/will to live kind. "So is this the. . ." I almost said "bad" one, but aren't they all, on some level, bad?

"Yes," she said quickly. "This is the traditional chemo. The lose your hair kind."

My heart sank. She meant the kind always depicted in movies where someone's rushing to the toilet to throw up, or looking like death warmed over.

"This would be an insurance policy, to increase your odds the cancer doesn't come back," the oncologist said.

But. . . wait.

"But she doesn't have cancer right now," my husband said. He hadn't yet gone in the white room, thank God. "She's cancer-free."

Which, of course. Why would you need chemo if you don't fucking have cancer?!

"Well, there's none we can measure, no," she said. "But if a single cell escaped. . .This is like an insurance policy."

Oh, God. A single drunk bitch could've stumbled in the Uber somehow, and we didn't even know?

"What if. . . what if I do nothing?" I asked. "Like, if I don't do chemo?"

"Probably somewhere around an 80% chance the cancer doesn't come back," my doctor said.

Oh, well, that sounded good, didn't it?

"And if I got the chemo?"

"More like 90% or more chance, the cancer doesn't come back."

Okay. Well, that sounded good. But also, a ten percent (ish) increase WITH the chemo? What's ten percent?

"So, let me get this straight. I'm going to poison my body. For three months, with follow-up immunotherapy treatments for nine months after that, for ten percent?" It was hard to feel like it was worth it. "So why would I do that? For just ten percent?"

"Well, because the cancer could come back, and if it does, it'll be metastasized; it will be stage four, and while we can treat it, we can't cure it, and it will kill you."

Well, fuck me.

I looked at my husband. What the hell? I needed an off-ramp. Maybe the cancer would come back in a decade. Maybe I didn't have to worry about this now. *If* the cancer came back. But what if that was when I was seventy? Eighty? Ninety?

I mean, did I really have to do this now? Hadn't I already given so much? Did I really need another battle right now? I imagined myself dipping out now, taking a break, pushing this decision down the road a couple of decades.

"Okay, so if one cell or so got loose. . . when would it come back?"

"Right, well, most of the time it comes back within a year. Two at most."

Fuck.

I thought about my youngest daughter—a sophomore in high school—and imagined her standing at my grave *before* she even graduated high school. I imagined my oldest—a junior— and how I might not even get to see *where* she went to college.

These were not milestones far into the future like weddings and babies. These were regular, run-of-the-mill milestones that I assumed I'd 100% be there for and never had any doubt I'd miss.

Unless I was dead.

Still, I wanted to bargain. "Couldn't I get the chemo later, though?"

Like, what if I tackled this next year?

My oncologist shook her head. "All the studies say you need it now. You've got a window, probably of about six weeks, but we'll need to do it now or you lose your window."

✧　✧　✧

The Fucking Window

It's rough when you're supposed to *voluntarily* choose chemo. Like, you don't necessarily *HAVE* to have it, but you probably should or else face death in a year.

Friends and family disagreed about the best course of action—everyone had their own opinions. My mom, who mistrusts medical professionals, felt the oncologist was exaggerating because that's what doctors do to protect themselves from malpractice and to make a whole bunch of money from treatments I may or may not need. My dad, the retired surgeon, took a simpler approach. "When it's Big C cancer, kid, don't mess around. Throw everything you've got at it when you have the chance."

All my organic friends felt chemo would be the worst thing I could do for my body and might even take years off my life. Other friends felt like I'd regret it forever if the cancer came back and I hadn't done everything I could to fight it.

My husband, PJ, simply said, "Your choice. I'll get behind whatever you choose. Just live, please."

Tons of voices argued in my head about it, and I'll be honest, my very first thought was: no fucking way.

It's not even the losing of my hair I worried about (though that's no fucking walk in the park), but it was the nausea and throwing up. I will do almost anything to avoid throwing up. I literally hate it more than anything. It's the worst. I know this isn't rational. Fears and phobias aren't rational, by definition.

So, I got a second opinion.

Get out of here, kid.

I didn't like my choices:

Go bald and be sick with a four-hour dose of poison to my system every single week for three months. . . or. . . possibly go into hospice before my youngest graduates high school.

Shit choices.

So I got a second opinion. I went to the premier muckity-muck director of impressive programs and writer of prominent research papers at the best hospital in downtown Chicago.

Dr. Muckity Muck was almost as old as my dad and had that same "rub some dirt on it" energy. His hair was entirely white. He was used to seeing strange and dire cases, women in stage four struggling to live, really complicated situations. Mine, however, was relatively straightforward.

"You can have the chemo or not have the chemo. I can tell you to do one thing or another, but you'll just hear what you want to hear, all patients do," he said in that jaded tone that told me he was already bored with my case. "But I'll tell you this. The chemo isn't as bad as you think it is. I have firefighters and police officers who get this treatment and go back to work. So you'll be fine."

The subtext was if a bald woman on chemo can rush into a burning building and save a baby, then I can sit at my keyboard and type out happily ever afters. Jesus, what the hell was wrong with me? Was a weak little cry baby?

He was almost annoyed with me, I'd say.

"Look, you could always try it. If you don't like it. . . you can quit."

It was then that I realized I'd been wringing my hands over what seemed like an impossible choice, so focused on the negatives and the fear, that I was missing the good news.

I was one of the lucky ones. I had a choice.

Plenty of other people don't get that. Plenty of people got the "the only way you can live is chemo" speech.

My case? Relatively straightforward, definitely treatable, and I could decide whether or not to have the chemotherapy. I could definitely try it and quit if I wanted. Dr. Muckity Muck's boredom with my case also underscored this fact: I could get treatment, not get treatment. He said, chances were, I'd probably be fine.

Also, his whole attitude screamed, "Get out of here, kid. Come back when you really have a problem."

This was what I needed. This sounds callous and awful, but this was exactly what my fuck-it Gen X sensibilities needed.

Now, he was right—that whatever he said, didn't really matter. I'd make my choice and either one would probably be fine (80% by doing nothing? Pretty good odds, no matter how you slice it). But he also laid a challenge out there, too.

Firefighters and police officers do it. What? Are you scared? You chicken? Bawk. Bawk. If you're so scared, you can always quit, crybaby.

It was that throwdown that eventually got me. My feral, drink-from-the-hose generation, that rode our bikes till dusk and worked out our disagreements without any adult intervention or counselor's anti-bullying program wanted to take the challenge. We wore our house keys around our necks and were fueled by Lucky Charms and sheer tenacity.

So, when someone tells me I'm not tough enough, I say *you're not tough enough*.

Also, I decided that I wanted to do everything I could *while* I could. If the cancer came back, I wanted to look at my kids, my husband, my family, and friends, telling them *I did everything I could do*. If the cancer came back, it wouldn't be on me.

Plus, Dr. Muckity Muck reminded me of my own agency. This wasn't a ride I couldn't get off of. I could quit at any time.

Everything you never wanted to know about chemo.

The masked nurse sat with us in the exam room and calmly explained how she was going to poison me every week for four hours for the next three months (plus two hours for immunotherapy). Nausea, hair loss, brittle nails, diarrhea. Check, check, check. Got it.

It's not really like the movies, she says. It's not like you're throwing up all the time. I mean, some people do, but then you'll have to let her know if that's the case.

What you really need to look out for is numb fingers and toes. That could be permanent.

Great.

I was used to cancer throwing shit grenades. I'd heard about the numb fingers and toes. All right.

"And chemotherapy often jumps starts menopause if you're not already in it," she adds. "So get ready for that."

Um. Great. Fantastic.

But. . . what about the weight loss? I'm expecting to be told to watch out. I'll drop twenty pounds in a flash, and then people will be worried, except I won't be worried because then I'll finally be at my post-first-baby, pre-second-baby weight. I'm looking forward to this. I've been stuffing my face with Christmas cookies because I've been telling myself, why not? I won't be able to eat anyway when they're pumping poison into my veins, so give it to me straight. Just how much weight am I going to lose?

"There won't be weight loss," she says. "In fact, there'll probably be weight gain."

"Weight gain?" I repeat these words because she has to be wrong. I've been secretly hoping that the Chemo diet might finally, *finally* take care of that extra ten (or 15 or 20) pounds I've been carrying around since COVID lockdown.

"Yes. Most people think you lose weight. But most gain weight." Partly because—surprise!—they pump you full of steroids before every dose.

What the Goddamn Fuck.

I'm supposed to go through chemo, lose my hair, get mouth sores, lose feeling in my fingers, and I don't even GET TO LOSE WEIGHT?!

What fresh hell is this?!

"So, wait. You *gain* weight? How much weight?"

"People will say they notice it."

Notice? I put on ten pounds during lockdown and didn't notice because I went months without putting on pants with a zipper and a button. I can gain a lot and not ever notice until someone takes a picture of me and posts it on Instagram, and then I'm like *Who the hell is she?!*

"Like a lot?" These are the most questions I've asked about *everything*, including permanent numbness in my toes, and the fact that I should wear ice booties if I don't want the numbness to be permanent.

"I mean, not fifty pounds or anything, but people notice it."

Okay, so not fifty pounds. But that could mean forty pounds. Easy. Shit.

"With the chemotherapy drug you're getting, people tend to gain weight. And have diarrhea."

I've got the runs *and* I gain weight? I don't understand. I'm in a dimension where nothing makes any goddamn sense.

You might be able to keep your hair if you don't mind freezing.

There are ways to try to keep your hair during chemo. It usually involves freezing your hair while you're having treatment. This means, essentially, wetting your hair and wearing a "freeze cap"—think an air-conditioned beanie that blows cold air on your already wet hair so that the chemo doesn't reach your hair follicles.

Women often choose this when they don't want the stress of losing their hair.

I had this option.

I turned it down.

Like everything with cancer treatment, there's a downside, and I, personally, just didn't want to deal with the downside. The freeze camp would add two hours to my treatment. That's right, *two hours*. That meant I'd spend a full workday—eight hours—at the cancer center every Friday.

Also, the cap only guaranteed keeping 65ish% of your hair, and I already had thin hair, so. . . huh? Did it even make sense? What if I went through the extra time and discomfort and *DIDN'T EVEN LIKE* the outcome?

Also, I already had to wear ice packs on my hands and feet because a side effect of my particular chemo treatment was nerve damage to my feet or hands. This could be permanent.

And I live in Chicago. I was getting chemo in the dead of winter, and the last thing I wanted to do was sit in a room with wet hair, with an air conditioner on my head AND ice mitts on my hands and feet. Might as well just go cannonball into the snowbank near the freeway. I don't like the cold that much, thank you.

Still, I don't judge anyone who uses the cap and wants to keep their hair.

Chemo was worse—and better—than I thought.

So, my understanding of cancer and chemotherapy treatment largely came from the movies:

Debora Winger dying of an unnamed cancer in *Terms of Endearment*; Star-Lord's sick, bald, white-as-a-ghost mom in *Guardians of the Galaxy*. And a host of made-for-TV-movies through the '80s and '90s.

You tell me chemo, and my mind immediately goes to all my hair falling out and *Exorcist*-style puking.

That's not what happened.

Here's the truth of *my* particular kind of chemo (and remember there are a billion different kinds, specifically tailor-made for different strains of cancer – my experience WILL NOT be your experience). Some people will get chemo and barely even feel it. Some people, no doubt, like those firefighters and police officers in Dr. Muckity Muck's office, they will get treatment and then pull on their uniforms the next day and go save the world.

How was Chemo better than I feared?

Well, for one thing, I wasn't puking my guts out all the time. My doctor prescribed two different kinds of anti-nausea medicine, both of which were amazing. My digestive system was thrown ALL out of whack, but I could still go out. I could still shop. I could still do things.

Dr. Muckity Muck was right: on most non-infusion days, I could work, cook, pick up the kids from school, and do my normal things just fine. I wasn't, actually, laid out in my bed in the ICU barely able to lift a cup of ice.

Yes, I felt fatigued, but quite honestly, what fifty-year-old woman with a full-time job and three kids in high school does NOT feel fatigued?

How was it worse?

My digestive system went haywire, and not in the puking my guts sense, because that would be cinematic and awesome. No—in the sense that everything supposed to be solid was liquid. I was running to the bathroom almost every single time after I ate, and often in between. (I've also heard the opposite is true of many chemo patients—constipation is a big one, too. So trust, your digestive track will be upset SOME way during this process.)

I had to cut out anything good to eat. This meant: no dairy (cheese! My fav!), or coffee (my whole identity), or spicy foods, or greasy foods. . . or anything you actually want to eat or drink. It was lean chicken, rice, and boiled vegetables for me for three months.

Also, no alcohol at all during chemo (and spoiler, everyone, barely any alcohol after either because alcohol does cause cancer).

I didn't gain weight during treatment; I lost it, so that first nurse got it wrong. To add insult to injury, the other nurses told me that I needed to keep my weight steady or the chemo wouldn't work as well as it should. Except I couldn't eat anything, so keeping up my weight was hard. I fooled them by lifting more weights and building muscle. I kept my weight similar even though I was losing fat.

My hair stayed much longer than I expected, but it also took much longer than I thought to come back. I lost my eyelashes AFTER I finished chemo. And the first peach fuzz didn't come back until nearly two months after the last dose. But—fun fact—it came back THICKER and curlier than before. Go figure.

During this phase of cancer treatment, I'll be honest with you, I felt I was spared dramatic Exorcist-style sickness, and instead, the small joys of life were taken from me.

I couldn't even enjoy my morning cup of coffee. This was the worst blow.

I LOVE coffee. I live for coffee. My kids and spouse buy me "I love coffee" themed merch and socks for all the holidays. My cabinet is stocked with "don't talk to me until I've had my morning coffee" themed mugs. Starbucks can't give me bonus stars fast enough. This was a true blow. Not just to my daily joys but to my whole freakin' identity. Who was I if I wasn't a "I run on coffee" person?

You're giving me tea? Fucking *hot tea*? Do I look like the British Royal Navy in the 1700s? Throw that shit in Boston harbor.

I realize now this sounds like First World Problems. Like, I had to sacrifice coffee temporarily to fight cancer? Yeah, well, it was a *blow*, okay? It was a sacrifice I never expected to have to make.

I couldn't enjoy going out to eat—because a) I was bald with no eyebrows and felt ugly and b) couldn't even enjoy any food on the menu, anyway, except the bread in the breadbasket (kindly hold the butter).

The withholding of small joys hurt more than I imagined it would.

This meant I just had to work harder to find small joys.

Instead of wine, I had to find probiotic soda and new fancy organic teas I liked.

Despite being able to eat almost nothing, I did find little things I ate with minimum side effects: an English Muffin (I guess the British are coming, after all) with apricot jam at the top of the list. There's nothing better than a warm English Muffin with jam in all the nooks and crannies. I could eat this with no stomach upset and this little gem hit my gratitude journal daily list more than once.

I could still enjoy a California roll and tamago sushi, and I did, often.

I discovered pickled ginger, ginger candies, and ginger ale did wonders for my stomach.

And I also discovered that the taunt of *I could quit anytime* just made me want to finish out the damn doses.

The first chemo infusion

I couldn't sleep well the night before my first chemo infusion. This would be a harbinger to come of what chemo would be like since I got a heaping dose of steroids with every infusion, which lit up my system like a coke bender, making it nearly impossible to sleep.

But I didn't know that then.

I was just an anxious wreck. My brain was telling my body I needed to do this to make sure I saw my daughters graduate high school, but my body was yelling, "Are we really just going to voluntarily *poison* ourselves? What the fuck?"

I was lucky in that, on my first session, I had the very kindest nurse. She'd had chemo herself. I will forever and always be grateful to this nurse and the universe for putting such an amazing caregiver in my path on my very first infusion day.

Chemo is both long and boring and terrifying. There's a whole lot of hurry up and wait. They have to mix up your toxic cocktail, and that takes a minute. Then they've got to get your line going—that's either through your chemo port or an IV – and all these things take time. The first time the nurse brought in the bag of poison, I noticed the toxic warning on it usually present in the labs of zombie movies.

"Why is the tubing and bag a different color than the saline bag?" PJ asks, noting the robin's egg blue packaging.

"It's specially reinforced plastic so the chemotherapy doesn't burn through the plastic," the technician tells us, matter-of-factly.

Great. I am getting Alien blood/acid/toxic nonsense pumped into the chemo port at the big vein above my heart (because, also, chemo will destroy smaller veins). Um. Yea?

This is decidedly unfair that I'm worried about chemo turning my insides into mush because, if *anyone* is going to do that, it's going to be me. With Tequila. And Gin. And all the dirty martinis and palomas I can handle.

Question: Does taking in poison make you immune to poison? Am I like the Dread Pirate Roberts in *The Princess*

Bride, suddenly immune to poison because I've taken small doses for twelve weeks? Is this how he did it?

Hmmm.

I'm getting this in my veins, y'all.

Then, the tech reminds us that my bodily fluids will be toxic for forty-eight hours. Literally. Like if PJ or anyone in my house is exposed to any of them (spit—whatever), he could get sick. I'm cautioned to keep the toilet seat down when flushing or risk sickening my family.

Yikes.

This does bring up the question: Does this make me an Alien?! Is my blood now acid? Am I going to take out a platoon of space marines? Maybe this is the real origin story of Alien. Ridley Scott, call me.

Your ass will burn.

I get the steroids first. The nurse kindly warns me that, if they push them too fast, my sphincter will constrict and my anus will feel like it's burning.

Cool. Cool. Cool.

Exactly what I wanted.

This seriously DID happen to me several times. I got nurses who gave it to me slow and ones that gave it to me just a bit too fast. And the fast ones?

You feel like you will definitely shit yourself. Or have. Or you've just got an enema of Frank's Red Hot sauce. Then, the feeling passes, and you're okay.

If this is happening to you—tell your nurses to slow their roll. Slow that drop. Nice and low and slooooooooow.

Steroids make your body stronger, but they also wire you up more than eight pots of coffee. I can't sleep the night of therapy. I'm buzzing, and I feel like all the nerves in my hands are buzzing.

THERE'S NO GOOD BOOK FOR THIS

My stepson jokes that I might get 'roid rage soon. He jokes that I need to hit the weights STAT and take advantage of them. My family makes me laugh and takes my mind off the terrible.

If you are lucky enough to live in a state where marijuana is legal, man GET you some. I would never have slept at all without some sleep gummies.

Spin the Wheel of Misfortune

The thing about chemo is that it's never the same way twice. You will desperately want to find a pattern in your treatment so you can anticipate and plan (on day one after an infusion, I'm tired, and on day two, I'm nauseous, etc.). You'll absolutely work hard to find something in the tea leaves, hoping your first or second or third infusion will give you an idea about what the others will be like, so you can plan for what it will be like.

But chemo doesn't come with any certainty whatsoever.

Having chemo is like spinning the wheel of misfortune to see what side effect you might get.

It's time to play. . .

Wheel! Of! Misfortune!

And here are the stars of our show. . . you and your infusion nurse!

I felt like every day I just spun the Wheel of Misfortune to see which side effect would be the biggest pain in my ass today: Diarrhea? Insomnia? Burning scalp? Horrible acne? Extreme fatigue? Brain fog? Splitting fingernails? Burnt tongue? Painfully dry vag? One of these annoying symptoms would be worse than the others, but I never knew which it would be from day to day, or even hour to hour. Sometimes, I'd work myself up and think—*Okay, the morning after infusion is the worst*, but then I'd be wrong that week and about two days later, after the steroids wore off, would be my worst day.

No week was exactly the same. I lost a whole bunch of hair one day and then kept the rest for a week or longer. At the end of chemo, I thought—*Oh, no more hair loss!* Then, I lost my eyelashes a week after I finished treatment. One day, I'd be sick as a dog and spend it all day on the toilet, sucking on ginger candies. The next day, I'd be starving and could eat a full meal and be totally fine.

This was when I started telling everyone that plans are simply an illusion.

"Want to go to dinner?" my friends would ask.

"We'll see," I'd say. "Right now, plans are an illusion."

"Could you come watch my track meet?" my daughter would say.

"I'll do my best. Plans are an illusion."

"Can we set a work meeting?"

You get the idea.

Plans. Are. An. Illusion.

In some ways, plans always were an illusion. We humans have always liked to put a film of certainty over a very, very uncertain world. But cancer—and chemo treatment in particular—really underscores this truth.

I'm not telling you this to scare you. For the *millionth* time, your experience might be 100% different from my experience. You may never see a Wheel of Misfortune. Maybe it's all awesome. And, great! I hope it is.

I'm not trying to discourage you from getting chemo, either. I personally think it's better if you can prepare, that's all. Not that any of us can really plan for anything.

Since life is what happens when you're busy making plans.

PJ gives the best pep talks.

Right about now, my husband and I started filming ourselves going to chemo. PJ suggested we do it, and I asked him to give me a pep talk.

On the first one, I felt ready to get a serious pep talk, a somber pep talk, the kind that would get me through the first treatment.

Instead, he started cheering his head off.

"Yeah!" he shouted, sounding like the little league soccer coach he was. "Let's go DO this!"

I laughed—genuinely—because I couldn't figure out why he was so excited to have me get poison injected into my veins.

"What? You asked for a pep talk," he said. "*That's* a pep talk!"

And it was.

And we kept doing them. Each one, goofier and sillier than the last. We lip-synced to ridiculous songs. We did all the things.

Laughter is good medicine.

Chemo makes you feel like your body is jail.

It's day three since the third round of chemo. The steroids have worn off, and now I'm left with the poison. I had a fitful night of sleep because there are still enough steroids to interfere with that. And, there are only two positions I can even sleep in these days that don't aggravate the port or the expanders. My nose is dry like a hard booger that can't be removed, the tip of my tongue feels perpetually burned, and I can't even drink a nice cup of coffee unless I want to spend the morning shitting my brains out.

I'm pouting right now because I had zero fun this weekend.

The things that usually brought me joy were tempered and dulled by my new (temporary) reality. I couldn't enjoy a fancy cocktail at dinner out Friday because no alcohol. I ordered the scallops and then worried they were undercooked (they weren't), but the worry sent me into a spiral of what happens if I do get food poison on chemo—do I die? The oncologist said bacteria is worse than viruses for my wrecked immune system, and it's what they worry about. And then there's the extra-supportive and tight sports bra I need to wear everywhere. It's uncomfortable, but discomfort is better than pain, which is what I feel when the bra is off and the expanders pull on my port so I make that trade-off. And the never-ending dry skin that feels like my face will crack and fall off, no matter how much moisturizer I slather on it.

The next night, the kids want a burger and cheese curds from Culver's, and that sounds good to me because, some-times, a good fast burger is just what you want. And it has protein, which everyone screams that I need. But after three bites of that burger, I'm running to the bathroom and I stay there for an hour. It wasn't even spicy. But because I have chemo brain fog, I forgot—I'm not supposed to have greasy food.

They mentioned that. I conveniently forgot. Greasy food is a big no-no, and now I know why.

And my amazing friends ping my phone. They ask me how I am, and it's touching and wonderful, except I also feel the need to lie, to be positive, tell them it's not that bad. They shouldn't worry. And it's not. I should be grateful it's not worse because I know it can be worse. It can always be worse. But I'm not feeling grateful. I'm feeling confined.

Later, I take a long, hot soak in the bath, but it's hard to get comfortable in there, because my one expander is on the move. It tugs at the chemo port, and everything hurts. I can't feel the hot water on my chest which is unnerving and weird, something I don't think I'll ever get used to. And then I get ready for bed, except I can't get comfortable because comfort seems like something far away that I might never have again.

And then I realize: I'm in jail.

I'm in jail, and the prison is my body.

The sentence is three months of intensive chemo, and then nine months of probationary immune-therapy. After I'm free, will I even remember how to enjoy anything anymore?

Life tries to steal your joy. Don't let it.

When I was small, around two and a half, I got a fever. A high fever of 103. I went to the emergency room because that's what you do when a toddler has a high fever like that, and doctors couldn't figure out what was wrong with me. The fever didn't break in a few days. It kept on. I was admitted to the hospital. The lining around my heart expanded, my joints swelled, and doctors worried about me. I was too little to understand what was happening, really, and I barely remember this time.

My dad, the orthopedic surgeon, diagnosed me before the other doctors did. Junior rheumatoid arthritis. This is an autoimmune disease where children get very high fevers, and their immune systems attack their own bodies. If left untreated, children's joints can be permanently damaged. Some are disfigured and can't walk or write. I went on a regiment of daily aspirin and physical therapy. The fevers would come and go, and Mom always told me that I was so little but so determined to keep playing. Sometimes, the fever would lay me out, but other times, I'd fight to keep playing—with my dolls or blocks or whatever I wanted to do.

"You always fought so hard for your joy," she told me.

Life tries to steal your joy in any number of ways. Through toxic people, through grief and death, through unfairness and meanness. Cancer, and chemo in particular, are joy suckers. They will try to steal your joy, even from the smallest of life events. You won't know how much you enjoyed a good shit until you're no longer able to accomplish one. You will discover for the first time there are many joys and satisfactions in life you simply took for granted.

Cancer—and chemo—will strip you of your complacency. It will show you ALL that you didn't appreciate enough before.

Chemo is a death by a thousand cuts. No one side effect typically is devastating, but altogether, they're the worst.

Burnt tongue, windburn face, brittle, peeling nails, nose so dry it hurts, floating nausea. Sudden trips to the bathroom. Fatigue. Tiredness.

Hair is falling out.

In big clumps. I make jokes because laughing is better than crying, and laughing at fear is the best way to neutralize it.

I make mustaches from the hair. A really big clump is a little pet mouse. If I can find joy in this, I truly can find joy in anything.

Also, your gray hairs will be the last to fall out.

Why? Because the gray hairs are tough-ass bitches with real-life experience, who won't be pushed around so easy.

Chemo and cancer will do their best to steal your joy.

This is when you have to fight hardest for the joys that remain. Sharing a laugh. Reading a book you love. Spending time with people who energize you.

Cling to the joys that remain. Be certain in the knowledge that other joys WILL return. Because they will.

The Silver Lining of Chemo

It's hard to imagine a silver lining of chemo. But there is one. It's putting YOU first. It's listening to your body and your spirit, what those things need from you in any given moment. Chemo won't let you push down your needs and ignore them (you WILL be running to the fucking bathroom sometimes, I guarantee).

You will HAVE to listen to your wants and needs, and you WILL need to meet them, or things will get a whole lot worse for you quickly. If you don't rest when you need to, your body will MAKE you rest.

You will learn (maybe for the first time) that self-care isn't bullshit. It's absolutely fucking essential. This isn't lighting a candle and getting a manicure (though it can include those things), it's all about essential things you need. Rest. Bland food that won't upset you. Moving your body and taking walks when you feel up to it. Avoiding toxic people and places.

This is a time to get in touch with what you need and learn how to ask for what you need—from your family, your boss, your friends. You will learn to set boundaries (maybe for the first time in your life) and you might decide you actually LIKE not having to do a bunch of shit you hate. You might decide that it's a good thing to do some serious self-care.

You will have to search harder than you ever had for joy in your life. The simple things you took for granted—eating, drinking, sleeping, even shitting—will be dulled, interrupted or ruined by chemo.

You will have to find NEW things to be excited about. You will also celebrate the time those mundane joys return to your life.

Pep talk #12:

Hey there, Warrior. You've been spending a lot of time in the bathroom lately. I know. You feel a slow death by a thousand cuts, and you've spun the wheel of misfortune so many times you just can't take it.

This is the time when you're going to dig deep. When you're going to find a well of strength and perseverance deep in you that will power you through this dark time. It starts with putting one foot in front of the other. It starts with doing the NEXT thing you have to do, whatever that is.

One step at a time.
One hour at a time.
One day at a time.

Little by little, you will get there, fueled by the amazing well of strength in YOU. You may have never had to dig this deep before, so you don't know how deep your well is. Trust me, it's fathomless. You'll be surprised yourself how deep your will to live goes. You have the strength. You have the grit. You have the determination. It's all in you.

Chapter Thirteen
The Boob Job No One Asked For

"I am not this hair, I am not this skin, I am the soul that lives within."

—Rumi

All the doctor visits had been fucking awful. They just were. But when it came to meeting with the plastic surgeon for reconstruction surgery, I thought, *Finally, a visit that won't be awful.* Maybe it might even be. . . fun? P.J. was definitely looking forward to this one. He thought maybe there'd be a catalog of boobs? Maybe a whole wall of implants we could weigh and hold up to the light, so we could pick the ones out we liked?

I don't know. I thought it would be. . . I mean at worst, informative. At best, hopeful? After all, I'd heard stories: *So and so who I knew got a double mastectomy and then she got double ds! She decided to TRADE UP, you know?*

So for many reasons, I thought the trip to the plastic surgeon would be fantastic. Fun. Lighthearted. I thought I'd fall into something called *Legally Medical* starring Reese Witherspoon, who would pop into the office with a pink stethoscope, all smiles and bubbly good cheer, and introduce me to the gravity-defying new boobs that would mean I'd never need to wear a bra again my entire life.

This was not what happened.

This was not the fun visit. Because I forgot this is fucking cancer and there are no fun visits.

PJ and I are sitting in the waiting room of the plastic surgeon, and we're cracking jokes because this is what we do. He jokes that this is the only appointment he's looking forward to, and we both joke that we're going to shop for new boobs like new tires.

"Could we just line up boobs in a row and let me squeeze them? That is the best way to find your new ones. It's scientific," he joked.

He is kidding, of course. He's told me this is 100% my decision. I could have no boobs, small boobs, big ones. . . he doesn't have a real opinion. His only requirement? "You've got to live. Do not leave me alone with these kids," he'd said often before. We had three teenagers at home and two twenty-somethings out in the wild. Two of the five were just learning to drive.

We're light-hearted this morning because this isn't the oncologist or the surgeon, people who had dropped bad news grenades in our lap so quickly we couldn't throw them away fast enough. The plastic surgeon isn't going to tell us about survival rates. We feel like we're in a safe space.

The nurse calls us in. She's soft-spoken and petite, and we sit in the exam room for maybe a minute or two before the doctor comes in. She's tall, lithe, and blond, but also, at the same time, not what I expected. I hadn't even really watched *Nip/Tuck*, but I guess I had a stereotype in my head of plastic surgeons: happy-go-lucky, party-hard people who'd be all perfect, with bright-white smiles.

But the doctor is thoughtful. Scientific. Knowledgeable. There's no pool party vibe here. There's a *I went to Stanford and always got an A+ in all the AP science courses, when you could barely grab a C.* This is good, I think. I wouldn't want *me* operating on *me*.

Yes, we'll be doing reconstruction. And then there are the buts:

Implants are the most common way to do reconstructions, but. . .

There has been controversy about them. They might leak. They might need to be replaced. My body might reject them. I might have other symptoms like lupus, headaches, joint pain, or any number of things women have complained of, but science has failed to prove a link to implants. Some discontinued implants with a non-smooth outer layer once caused Leukemia.[39] But they don't use those anymore.

I'll have to decide silicon vs. saline.

Saline if it leaks, will just be absorbed by my body, but because it's saline, when I jog or move quickly, there might be sloshing sounds.

Sloshing!

What the holy hell?

Silicon was banned for years, but then brought back because scientists think it's safe now. However if I get silicone ones, there's no way to tell if there's a leak or break except by getting regular MRIs.

Both are foreign bodies, not natural to my own. And I won't have any of my own breast tissue around them, like women who choose to get implants. I'll just have skin covering the bag. They might show through my skin when I'm naked, in the form of odd wrinkling.

Wrinkling!!

What the hell is *odd* wrinkling…?

They might get hard calcifications around them over time. That you can feel.

---

[39] **Bilateral breast implant associated chronic lymphocytic leukemia/small lymphocytic lymphoma (CLL/SLL): A case report**, May 2020, National Institute of Health.

Oh, and if you get radiation, then you might not even be able to get implants at all because of the weird scars and. . . Well, it just might not work.

OR. . .

I could use fat from my own body. My abdomen. Be cut open from hip to hip, have fat removed from down there, and then put where my chest is. I'd have to have veins tied from my hip to my chest to get blood flow there.

This is obviously a more complex surgery and requires a longer recoup period and multiple scars. Well, so long, bikini.

Not that I ever really planned to wear a bikini, but I'd like to imagine one day I would.

I don't have a lot of fat on the abdomen, so the new boobs might even be smaller (!) than the ones I have now. But they'll "feel" natural. Fucking SMALLER boobs. Are you kidding me?!

Bonus: they won't slosh.

When I get my double mastectomy, they'll weigh what they take out. So they can put roughly the same amount back in.

I'll be weighed. Like. . . what? Like a bunch of grapes on a grocery store scale? I don't know. This is all seemingly suddenly absolutely awful.

But the bad news keeps coming.

And with any procedure, we'll have to worry about skin necropolis. Skin dying over the implant or the new fatty tissue, which might mean multiple surgeries to correct because who wants zombie boobs? *But you know what? We'll probably have cadaver skin that we'll graft to your chest anyway, so. . .*

I guess I will have zombie boobs anyway.

And I'm feeling a whole hell of a lot of. . . this is not Disney World at all. I want to get the hell out of here.

This isn't a consolation prize. This is a new nightmare I've fallen into. A nightmare within a nightmare. Why can't I wake up? Why?

"Do you know where you're leaning?" the doctor asks me. "Implants or. . ."

I know where I'm leaning.

I'm leaning toward: not this.

I don't want this.

I don't want any of this.

I don't want curtain one or two.

I don't want it.

I don't want any of it.

Or maybe you don't get reconstruction at all.

I was chatting with an oncologist I met at a party. I'd already had the double mastectomy and the chemo, and I'd also had the implants (I went with saline.—Spoiler, there's odd wrinkling that I don't think I'll ever get used to, but no sloshing—so far.), and I was cancer free and healed—mostly.

"I have a plastic surgeon who tells me all the time that, if she ever got cancer, she'd never do reconstruction," the oncologist tells me.

"Why?" I ask.

"Too many things that can go wrong. Too many ways it doesn't work out. They almost never look like people want them to look."

"But, she's a plastic surgeon. . ."

"I *know*, and she tells her patients: don't do this. It won't turn out like you like. But they do it anyway." The oncologist shrugs. "She tells me if *I* ever had breast cancer and needed a double mastectomy *not* to get reconstruction at all."

Some women are fine without boobs.

My mom tells me that, when she announces to her bible study group that her daughter has breast cancer, a bunch of other women let her know they'd had breast cancer, too. One woman said she'd even had a single mastectomy but never had reconstruction on that side. She opted for a prosthetic that she wore in her bra.

"I never even knew," Mom said. "So, see? You have options."

I thought I wasn't vain.

But then someone wanted to cut my boobs off and I had the option of going without—and I just didn't want to. I'd spent my adolescence stuffing bras, so I didn't really feel like doing that as an adult.

I also think—I'm fifty. I want to go to the beach still. I want to be able to wear V-neck sweaters. I don't know. . . I didn't want to look flat-chested. I'd been close enough to that my whole life.

So, I opted for the implants.

Saline.

And hoped I wouldn't slosh.

Expanding the Expanders

Right after the mastectomy, I got expanders inserted (read: sewn to my muscles). Expanders have a hard, round base and a silicon pocket that's deflated but has a small hole on top that can be accessed by a needle.

They're flat at first, and after I headed back to my plastic surgeon's office they got poked with a giant needle and filled up with saline. That's a big old needle to the boob, to get that saline in there. But I no longer could feel the skin there—so, shrug? Then, when I reached the size I wanted, the idea was to stop and then get my permanent implants put in. I couldn't wait because the iron bra of the expanders just sucked.

"Will my permanent implants be like this?" I asked, worried.

"Oh, no, no. They'll be much more comfortable. Nothing like this," the nurse assured me.

I couldn't sleep on my stomach (pain) or back (also pain) so the only thing that I could do was balance on my side propped up by pillows.

Then, one of them broke loose. The stitching snapped and one went rolling off to the right beneath my skin. I know this because it was obvious anytime I looked in the mirror. And also because the hole in the implant was encased by a plastic disc, which before had been steadfastly on the upper part of the placeholder boob, and now was spinning around up—down—sideways. So this meant I now had to wear a bra—the iron bra—24/7 so that I didn't gouge extra space under my armpit and the new, permanent implant wouldn't sink there, where it shouldn't be.

Even worse, my oncologist broke the news that the invasive tumor was slightly bigger than they thought. That meant my oncologist thought I needed chemo, so instead of having reconstruction surgery in six weeks like I planned, it would be in nine months instead (because spoiler—you can't have surgery while you're going through chemo, what with your weakened body and gutted immune system).

I went from having to wear the iron bra for six weeks—to NINE FUCKING MONTHS.

It was torture.

I was beginning to worry that the permanent implants would be just as uncomfortable, despite the nurse assuring me they're night and day. (I can attest—they are FAR more comfortable. Not perfect, not your real boobs, but MUCH better than the expanders.)

As I struggled to sleep because I simply could not get comfortable with the iron bra on, one friend thought they'd cheer me up by complimenting me on the size of them.

"Look at how magnificent they are!" she declared.

She meant well.

It's just hard to admit I really didn't care what they looked like. They were torture. Like more than the usual torture of stiletto heels, and I wear those only because I know I can eventually take them off.

Can I touch them?

After I got rid of the expanders and got my final implants, I'm at a friend's birthday party and a mutual friend tells me her husband wants to touch my new implants.

"He's never felt implants before," she says. "He's been talking about it a lot."

Later, he tells me this himself. "I've never felt implants before." Insert wiggle of eyebrows here.

They maybe had had too much wine.

And yet. . . other friends ask the same thing. "You are going to let me touch them, aren't you?" one friend insists.

You'd be surprised how often people just ask.

It was the same when I was pregnant. People wanted to touch my belly.

This might happen to you as well, so just be prepared.

You might ADORE your new boobs. You might want to flaunt them. Hell, you might ask perfect strangers at the grocery store to squeeze them instead of the cantaloupes.

That's not how I feel about mine.

The thing is: if I wanted implants, I would've gotten them by now.

I never wanted them.

My new slightly larger than C boobs are perfectly round and somewhat perky, but they are not mine. I feel them all the time and not in a natural way. I can't sleep on my stomach because it feels weird, and I have an absurd worry I'm going to pop them. They DO wrinkle—most especially when they're out of a bra—because the only layer between the implant and me is a very thin layer of donor/my skin and so I'm always a little anxious about them because they could misbehave at any time.

I'm 100% aware every single time I look in the mirror that I'm carrying around two saline bags in my chest. I never, ever forget this. They do not feel or act like real boobs.

They also feel weird when I jog sometimes (though, thankfully, they don't slosh—or hell, maybe they do, but I can't hear them with my earbuds in). They feel strange when I sleep on my stomach and also when people hug me—because I'm definitely aware I'm carrying around two Ziploc bags of saline in my chest cavity.

The breast surgeon saved my nipples, but I've lost all feeling in them; so if you grab my boob, I feel nothing. It might be tantalizing for the grabber but for me? The nerve endings are dead. It's like being poked through a comforter and a down jacket.

They look fine in clothes, but I don't wear plunging necklines or V-necks because I've got chemo port scars and. . . Remember that the skin wrinkles in weird ways? That is 100% not sexy.

"Oh. You don't like your new boobs?" One of my oldest friends is so sad for me.

I've made peace with my new boobs, but if I could wave a magic wand and get my old boobs back, the ones that I could feel, the ones that were natural, that don't wrinkle—but just healthy this time? I would.

All that said, I'm glad I have them.

I never felt so out of sorts as I did after the double mastectomy, having to look down at my Frankenstein scars and flat chest. I deliberately didn't look at those scars unless I had to, and the nurse and my husband reminded me at every stage that was temporary.

The bad ass women who DON'T get replacement boobs, I salute you. You're fucking brave bitches, and I love you.

I'm glad for the fake boobs, for the placeholders, so I don't have to stuff my bra. I also know it could be so much worse. The reconstruction could've gone terribly wrong, and it didn't. I'm lucky. But the implants aren't something I celebrate. They are more something I tolerate.

You may be different, of course. You may LOVE your new boobs.

Everyone experiences this different. Every journey is different. You may love this part of your journey.

Get new boobs—don't—the choice is yours.

The point of this chapter is to tell you that unfortunately, most of the time, reconstruction isn't the fun part of breast cancer. It's just not.

It's another serious surgery with potentially serious consequences. It may be painful and then they may not look like you want, and they probably won't, because they're not REAL. They don't even have a layer of REALness around them. They are saline or silicone bags of plastic. They are not and never will be real boobs.

Reconstruction CAN have good results. Now that I've come to accept they are not, nor ever will be real, I can still be glad I can fill out a sweater without worrying. In a bra, they look very nice. If faced with the same decision, I probably would've done the exact same thing.

You can make the same or a different choice. You can get multiple surgeries and use your own fat (I really hate the idea of anyone cutting on me, and so I just wanted to keep the incisions to a minimum), but plenty of people choose that option.

This is a deeply personal decision that only you can make.

The new boobs aren't your old ones. They're different. That's all.

Pep talk #13:

Hey, friend. You thought reconstruction would be the fun part until you were rudely reminded there is no fun part about cancer.

That's okay.

You will walk through the flames of this trying time, and you will emerge a phoenix from the ashes. You will rise a new, stronger, more resilient you. You will emerge looking different, that's true, but you will be EVEN MORE beautiful than you are now.

Whether you get new boobs or not, your beauty will shine from inside you. From the well of strength and resilience in you. No, you don't look like you used to. You'll be better. Stronger in all the ways that matter.

You will know that beauty isn't skin deep. Beauty, real beauty, comes from the soul, the unique light that is you.

Chapter Fourteen

Avoid Soul-Crushing Debt—If the Cancer Doesn't Kill You, the Debt Might. How to Make It All Work.

"I have cancer. Cancer doesn't have me."

—Marco Calderon

Most people think their health insurance is great because they've never had to use it. Once you get a diagnosis, you may find your insurance actually sucks.

Indeed.

Okay. Deep breaths.

For those of you who skipped "Chapter Six: Not all Doctors are Good" then quick recap: America's healthcare system is the most expensive in the world and delivers mid results at best. Millions of people delay life-saving diagnostic care because they don't have healthcare and can't afford it, and then when they finally do find the cancer, it's Stage Two or worse. And for women of color in this country? Good lord, don't get me started.

Even if you do have healthcare, you might have signed up for a budget plan, because when you're healthy, paying 30 or 40% of your medical costs doesn't seem like that big a deal. Except that the average cancer treatment costs well over six figures.

Medical bills remain the number one reason people in America declare bankruptcy for good reason. Medical care is expensive, and we live in a country that doesn't believe life-saving care is a right, not a privilege. No matter where you fall on the political spectrum, when you're dealt a cancer diagnosis and you have no insurance, you start believing maybe Bernie Sanders was right after all.

Cancer doesn't care if you're rich or poor. It strikes evenly, but if you're poor, then you feel like you're being held hostage. You're paying a ransom on your life, and it's every damn medical bill that slips into your mailbox. Plenty of women struggling to pay for breast cancer treatment, put off appointments or take less of their medications to save money, which is tragic.[40]

Also, you might think you've got badass insurance because you've never been sick. And now suddenly that same insurance is denying your claim (Do you need another biopsy? Are you really sick, or are you faking it, Karen?). You might find yourself finally paying attention to that Maximum Out of Pocket Number or Deductible and realize that you actually don't have that kind of cash lying around.

Here's the good news: breast cancer is stupidly common. Breast cancer survivors and their families are badass mothers, who have spent their lives raising money for the cause. There are resources out there for you.

Use them.

Let's talk about what you can do now to make sure you're not spending the last days of treatment sleeping beneath a highway overpass.

The top reason people declare bankruptcy is medical bills.
So tell me again about how great our healthcare system is.

When you've got to decide whether you get evicted or get life-saving treatment, tell me again how we live in the greatest country in the world?

---

[40] Covering Cost of Care, BreastCancer.org.

One in ten Americans has outstanding medical debt. More than half a million families file bankruptcy every year because of medical bills—that's 59% of all bankruptcies. Also, fun fact, France has ZERO medical bankruptcies.[41]

Even if you have health insurance, you're going to have to meet your deductible, and you WILL meet your out-of-pocket costs, and for many families, those numbers are five digits.[42] If you don't have health insurance, know that your breast cancer diagnosis might cost anywhere from $20,000 on the low end, to well over $100,000 on the high end.

Chemo can cost several thousand dollars a round. Cases can be different, and surgeries can have complications.

And now might be the very first time you ever pay attention to your Out-of-Pocket Maximum. You might have thought $18,000 for a family seemed low when you signed up for your plan, and now you've got to come up with $18,000—cash.

Our healthcare system doesn't work for most of us.

If you, like my dental hygienist, were diagnosed with breast cancer right before she got a new job before her insurance kicked in, you're not alone.

When I was diagnosed with breast cancer, my husband had just launched his own franchise logistics business. In my professional life, I'd rarely been lucky enough for corporate health insurance because I'm a freelance writer and rarely qualified for benefits. I'd been a regular user of the Healthcare Marketplace (Affordable Healthcare Act).

---

[41] "Medical Bankruptcies Statistics," *Balancing Everything*, February 2, 2024.
[42] Jen Uscher, "Special Report: The Cost of Breast Cancer Care," BreastCancer.org.

P.J. joked when we got married in 2018 that I was marrying him for his corporate healthcare benefits.

But then he decided to get off the corporate train and we were on COBRA. That was fine because health insurance is something no one thinks about until they actually need it.

I went to get a mammogram because I knew the COBRA was running out. I never expected to get diagnosed with cancer.

And did I mention the COBRA was RUNNING OUT?

Cancer is a ticking bomb. Delay too long and Stage I becomes Stage II. It becomes more entrenched in your body, and that messy bitch gets an uber. . . Suddenly your outcomes start to look bleaker and bleaker. And, by the way, the treatment gets more and more expensive.

Because you're waiting on fucking insurance? Seriously?

I found myself in real trouble after my diagnosis. I was wondering if we'd have to get a second mortgage on the house to pay for treatment.

Well, thank the universe or God or whomever you pray to, that I had an amazing insurance agent friend who'd saved me once before.

Twelve years ago, I was a single, divorced mom to two beautiful girls, and my youngest developed a peanut allergy. We'd skated by on bare-minimum freelance health insurance (this was before the Affordable Care Act). When she had a serious reaction and I found myself calling an ambulance, I was dealing with a multiple thousand (!) dollar bill I had no idea how I would pay back (turns out slowly, over time, after negotiating with the hospital).

This told me I needed better health insurance, and I needed it fast. Another freelancer and a dear friend who was also queen of the gig-economy referred me to Mark Gurda at Castle Group. I owned my own company, but it simply had an employee of one. he was used to dealing with bigger corporations, but he still helped me find insurance to help pay for my daughter's treatments.

Here again, I reached out to him, and here again—he saved us.

Thankfully, with my husband's small company, if he brought me on as a full-time employee (which I was already doing behind-the-scenes work for free so paying me made sense), then we'd have enough employees to get our own medical plans. We picked the most expensive (but also the most comprehensive one).

The downside was twofold: he couldn't really afford to pay me a salary, and we hadn't planned to add health insurance for all employees yet. Health insurance ended up costing us about $3,000 a month, plus my salary, and I now had two maximum out-of-pockets and two deductibles to deal with in one year.

Cancer is an expensive bitch, and pretty soon, those costs seemed small compared to the bills I saw coming in the mail.

Don't freak out. Yet.

Do not avoid getting the tests or treatments because you're worried about the cost. This is not the time to go bargain shopping.

You're in the middle of some horrible choices: delay care until it's cheaper, or you figure out how to pay for it and risk that your cancer spreads, getting harder to treat.

Look, as scary as it is to pull the trigger and rake up credit card debt, or get a home equity loan, or all the other horrible options to get the care you need NOW, I'm going to tell you this:

The earlier you treat the cancer, the cheaper the care will be.

You are NOT saving money by waiting. And you could be risking your life by waiting.

Also, fun fact, sometimes you might not get the bill right away. It might come in a couple of weeks, or even months later, and by then, maybe you've got a way to pay. Get the test first. Get the treatment first. Worry about how you will pay for it later.

You have options.

There are dozens and dozens of charities that can help with costs. There's the healthcare marketplace (for now) that might let you enroll in healthcare while you figure everything else out. Also, you CAN negotiate with hospitals and doctors if you don't have health insurance. Did you know if you don't have insurance that hospitals and healthcare networks often will knock off a percentage (maybe even a quarter or a third) of your bill right off the top? Call them. Talk to them. You'll be surprised.

You also can take an emergency withdrawal or loan from your 401k with minimum penalties to pay for care. You can start a GoFundMe, of course. And there are a ton of resources out there, too.

So, how do you start getting your financial plan together?

First thing's first—start making your paper trail.

Keep every invoice and every bit of paperwork you get about your diagnosis and treatment. Start a folder and keep EVERYTHING. You might be tempted to burn the bills you get or stuff them in the trash because they're so terrifying, but you need to keep them. All of them.

Why? Because you may find a nonprofit program that will reimburse some of your costs. You may be able to negotiate certain services down from the hospital. You may have to fight your current insurance about what they pay.

You need a paper trail because you aren't just going to have to fight cancer; you may have to fight a whole lot of pencil-pushing bureaucrats. They may want to drain your will to live more than the tumor growing inside you, but you've got this. Arm yourself with the proper weapons.

Get financial help and advice.
Here's the good news about having a cancer that affects 1 in 8 women in America. There ARE actually resources designed to help you. You're not the first woman to arrive at a cancer center with subpar or no insurance. This happens ALL the time (see: shitty American healthcare system).

This is NOT something to be embarrassed about.

I'm going to say this once: You deserve to live. You deserve care. It doesn't matter if you don't have a cushy corporate job with benefits or were trying to save a few dollars this year by opting out of health benefits. It doesn't matter that you didn't save up an emergency fund like your brother nagged you to do, and now you're in trouble. It doesn't matter if you've been desperately stringing together gigs like Uber and Instacart and you can barely pay your utilities.

You DESERVE care.

You DESERVE to live.

Getting treatment for cancer isn't eating caviar on a fucking mega yacht, so don't treat it like a splurge or something "only rich people" are allowed to have.

You deserve it, too. This isn't charity. It's the battle of your fucking life.

If you're not rich or loaded up with an amazing healthcare plan, then it'll take some hustle. But you're used to that.

So, let's make this shit happen.

Assess what you actually do have.

Have insurance? Read the fine print.

Figure out exactly what they owe you. This could take some doing, and it could take help because healthcare contracts are deliberately hard to understand.

Have a 401k? Does your spouse? You can take a hardship loan.

If you do have retirement savings, you can take an emergency loan to pay for your (or your spouse's) healthcare costs without extra penalty. I know we're told never to touch our retirement savings, but do not pinch pennies here. Worry about how you'll make up that savings later, my friend. Meeting your retirement goals won't help you if you don't live to see retirement.

Talk to the finance experts.

You can start with the finance office of your hospital or healthcare network. Hey—surprise!—doctors and hospitals like to be paid. And if they're really on it, they might even assign you to a specific person. They'll likely have a designated group within their finance department designed to help you figure out how to pay for your care. You can start there. Don't be afraid to reach out. They probably have staff members whose sole job is to help you find resources because—again – they like to be paid.

They might direct you to state-funded organizations or nonprofits that can help you. They might have advice on where to get insurance (like the Affordable Care Act, AKA Obamacare).

Need more help? Try:

Triage Cancer's Legal and Financial Navigation Program. They give free legal and financial advice to cancer patients and their caregivers.

The Patient Advocate Foundation (PAF) provides case management and can pay for treatment and living expenses. They help patients understand their employment/medical benefits and rights.

Need more resources? Search the **Cancer Financial Assistance Coalition**'s database of organizations who can help or check out BreastCancer.org.[43]

Also, almost all drug companies have financial assistance programs. See

https://www.pparx.org

https://youngsurvival.org/directory/partnership-for-prescription-assistance-pparx

If you don't have insurance, look into how you can get some.[44]

Your best first step might be to talk to an insurance agent, like I did. But here's an overview of what's available to you:

Corporate Health Insurance
We know these are the benefits through our jobs or our spouse's jobs. Most of these benefits only allow changes at certain times of the year or for a special life change, like marriage.

The Affordable Care Act
This also has special enrollment periods, but these benefits aren't linked to a job. The ACA (Heathcare.gov) requires its plans to cover mammograms and breast cancer treatment. This Act also made denial of care from pre-existing conditions (congrats—

[43] Jen Uscher, Farida Rangwala, "Charitable Resources for People Diagnosed with Breast Cancer," BreastCancer.org.
[44] Tanya Feke, MD, "A Breakdown of Breast Cancer Insurance Coverage," Very Well Health, November 19, 2024.

cancer is the pre-existing condition of a lifetime!) illegal.

Medicaid
This is state-funded insurance largely for folks who can't afford it. You can enroll in this at any time, but there are a few hoops to jump through to qualify.

Medicare
If you're over sixty-five, you're probably well acquainted with Medicare. Medicare, however, has limits to coverage.[45]

The State Health Insurance Assistance Program offers individual counseling and help for navigating Medicare.

Step Four: Reach out to nonprofit organizations. There are grants out there. Go get 'em.

- **Susan G. Komen's Komen Financial Assistance Program** can help with daily living expenses such as rent, utilities, childcare, or elder care, as well as medical equipment and home healthcare.
- **The Pink Fund** has a 90-day grant program to cover the cost-of-living expenses for people in active treatment.
- **Living Beyond Breast Cancer Fund** gives out need-based grants.
- **Cancer and Careers** also gives out grants.
- **United Breast Cancer Foundation** gives grants to support people who are receiving treatment for breast cancer or who have been in remission for three years.

---

[45] "What Medicare Covers," medicare.gov/publications/11931-medicare-coverage-of-cancer-treatment-services.pdf.

- **The Patient Advocate Foundation (PAF)** has a co-pay relief fund for those who quality.
- **Infinite Strength** can help you cover rent or your mortgage for six months for single parents.
- **Allyson Whitney Foundation** offers Life Interrupted Grants of $500 to $1,500 to young adults diagnosed with breast cancer who are in active treatment.

I was not kidding—there are plenty of organizations and people out there who can help you. LET them. This is just the tip of the iceberg. You are not alone in this.

And again—remember, when you're worried about how to pay for this, you might already jump ahead to bankruptcy, losing your job, or all the other horrible outcomes, but that's also fear talking. Remember that fear is turbulence, it's not the plane crashing. You may not have to declare bankruptcy. You might not have to drain your 401k or max out your credit cards. Or, hear me out, even if you do—YOU'LL BE ALIVE AND NOT DEAD. Okay? So, get the care.

The whole trick in surviving this process is to keep your priorities straight—and keep your eye on the prize. Your first priority is fighting the cancer.

Pep talk #14:
Hi, Soldier. Money woes getting you down? You might feel like giving up. You might feel like hope is lost.

It's not lost. It's just hard to see right now.

There are people out there wanting to help you. They only need you to find them. And you won't find them if you give up.

Don't give up. Don't skimp on care because you're worried about the bill.

Help is on the way. Help is waiting. Go find it. The universe wants you to be better, and it's colluding with others to give you a path through this. It's working behind the scenes, conspiring to find you a path.

Keep looking. You'll find the path.

Chapter Fifteen

The Cancer Card Trumps All—
Play that Card Early and Often

"Cancer is a word, not a sentence."

—John Diamond

There's only one upside to cancer.

There are a lot of people who tell you that you'll find a silver lining in all this. Maybe you could start a charity, or form a support group, or raise thousands of dollars for cancer research. And, sure, you could do those things.

But as far as I'm concerned, there's only one upside to cancer.

It's the excuse you need to get out of absolutely anything.

It is your get-out-of-jail-free card. Use it!

I mean, you've got to deal with the terror, the looming mortality, the side effects of all the treatments and the surgeries, and the ginormous fucking bill. So play that cancer card. Play it until it's worn out.

It's the best built-in excuse for a "no" you'll ever have. Seriously. Tell me what you say to someone who tells you, "I'd really love to. . . X. Y. or Z. But I'm sorry. I've got breast cancer. I've got to focus on getting well."

What is the comeback to that? THERE IS NONE.

There's simply: "Oh, my God. I hope you feel better soon. Do not worry about a thing. We got X, Y, and Z."

You need someone to volunteer to sell concessions at the school football game? Sorry! Cancer.

You need someone to fundraise for your work charity? Sorry! Cancer.

Hey, old roommate from college I can't stand. You're in town and want to grab dinner so you can suck me into a new Ponzi scheme? Sorry! Cancer.

Hey, want to teach a course on creative writing, even though you hate talking in front of people? Sorry! Cancer.

Hey, you want to pick up the extra slack at work or this freelance assignment that's going to be an absolute drag and will make me want to poke out your own eyes with a pen? Sorry! Cancer.

Want to host the holidays this year? Sorry! Can't. Cancer.

Any chance you want to spend way too much money to visit friends you aren't even close to because they planned a trip without you and only thought of inviting you at the last minute? Sorry! Cancer.

Want to be in my wedding even though I know you talk about me behind my back? Nope! Sorry, Cancer.

Want to cook something from scratch for the school bake-off? Sorry! Cancer.

Your old boss wants to offer you a new job at the company you hated and vowed never to return to? Sorry! Cancer.

Hey, want to grab coffee with the neighbor that you secretly hate because she says mean, passive-aggressive things about the state of your yard? Sorry! Cancer.

That aunt by marriage who loves to gossip is in town and you'd been planning a quiet night alone, nose buried in a book, or in a bubble bath. With wine. You should meet her because she's only here every freakin' quarter. Nope! Sorry. Cancer.

Hey, that old coworker who talks too loud, has the exact opposite politics as you, and likes to rant about the presidential election *in June* at the top of his voice in a crowded environment? Well, he wants to get drinks. Sorry! Nope. Cancer.

It's the best built-in excuse, but the *reason* it's the best built-in excuse is because you don't have time for any other bullshit. You don't have the energy. You don't have the focus, either. Every bit of you will be dealing with the psychological and physical blows cancer is about to rain down on you.

Play the cancer card. Do not be shy. Cancer blew up your life, so the least it owes you in return is the perfect excuse to get out of lunch with the coworkers you hate.

It's not even *bad* to play the cancer card. It's a good thing.

Because the one thing cancer shows you is that you simply do not have the time or energy for any bullshit right now.

You need every bit of strength to get through what's about to happen, and you can't be psychically drained by meaningless, people-pleasing activities designed to suck your will to live. You need ALL your will to live right now. That means avoiding negative people and situations.

This doesn't mean you can't enjoy the upside. That trip to the in-laws? The boring dinner with your boss? The extra volunteer activities? The expensive trips with college friends, who make more money than you, but keep inviting you to Vail anyway? All of the bullshit you've been saying a tepid yes to because you couldn't figure out how to say no without hurting everyone else's feelings?

Well, now you won't.

Now, no one can tell you you're being selfish.

YOU HAVE FUCKING CANCER.

And that's enough bullshit for anyone to deal with.

So, you're playing the cancer card, and you've broken the news to people. Now let's talk about what you're going to do next.

Say no to everything. You will find your True No faster than ever. Dare someone to try to pull you into a church meeting. Say no. Say it often. Use the Cancer Card. Everything about this sucks, except that you never have to go to that catty bitch's neighborhood party ever again if you don't want to. You don't have to see your braggy cousin's new kitchen. You don't have to drive halfway across the country to visit your in-laws who will ask you if you've gained weight and why haven't you gotten that promotion yet.

Oh, the Cancer Card is wonderful. Use it. You'll need the time to rest and recuperate. You'll need to say no to all those soul-draining exercises because you'll need all the energy you need for the fight ahead.

The Beauty of No

We're trained all of our lives, as women, to be accommodating. To smile. To be good Helpers. To say yes. If we don't do these things, we're difficult, aggressive, bitchy. Most of us suffer from the Disease to Please.

But cancer frees you from societal expectations to a certain degree. The sad part is we had the power to say no THE WHOLE TIME, and it takes something like a deadly cancer to give some of us (me) the excuse to actually say it guilt free. That's the thing. I said no ALL the time, to ALL kinds of things, and felt ZERO guilt. It was. . .magnificent.

Say no.

Say it loud!

Draw those boundaries in Sharpie so they're never erased.

It's a glorious feeling. Wonderful. Amazing.

But what will people think about me?

You say no to your passive-aggressive neighbor's housewarming because you don't feel like standing in her new kitchen while she brags for two hours about her Viking stove.

You say no. You stay home and have an amazing evening on your couch watching trash TV and eating popcorn, feeling reenergized because you don't have to listen to her brag and flex about how that damn oven was flown in from halfway across the world. In a special fucking gold helicopter accompanied by flocks of white doves or some such nonsense.

You say no.

And you know what you'll discover?

The world does not fucking end. People do not gossip about how selfish/awful/problematic you are. And even if they do—so what? They're shallow, horrible people who like to kick a person when they're down. When they have CANCER.

The best people in your life will say no for you.

And here's something else that's interesting: other people will say no for you. The very best people in your life will step in and take the "volunteer to send a fundraising email to your alumni class" task for you. They'll say things like, "You've got breast cancer and you don't have time for this shit," and they'll pick up the slack.

It's awesome and amazing.

These people will jump in front of mundane work tasks for you—LET them. When you're well (and you will be well), you can do the same for someone else who is suffering.

I had friends who would invite me to dinner, and because they knew I was such a pleaser at heart, they'd also say, "It's okay to say no."

Cancer is using you every day. Return the favor.

My daughter fretted about what to write about for her college essay. Colleges these days are just so competitive and how could she possibly stand out?

When I got breast cancer, it became a disease the entire family had to deal with. It's scary when your mother falls prey to something like this. I knew it would be stressful. But because it's me, I did crack a joke:

"Hey, what are you sad for? I just gave you the very *best* topic for your college essay. You're welcome."

She laughed as she sniffed back tears.

It sounds audacious and horrible. Take advantage of cancer?

Fuck, yes, take advantage of cancer.

Do you think it cares at all? YOU are suffering on every level: mentally, physically, and spiritually. Why not use cancer to your advantage when you can? Want to die a lonely martyr?

No, you don't.

And you also don't want to go to your sister-in-law's Mary Kay party. So don't.

You'll Need Your Strength

The hard truth is that you can't pitter away your strength doing things that suck you dry. You're going to need every ounce of fight in you for cancer, not for passive-aggressive comments from in-laws or neighbors. You can't afford to share your energy with fundraisers or toxic people (see Chapter Seventeen: Cut Out Toxic People—You Can Only Deal with One Malignant Asshole at a Time, and Right Now That's Cancer) because right now you've got to be laser-focused on getting well.

And you've got to maintain whatever works for you: blinding positivity, grinding anger, sarcasm—whatever powers you through tough times. I'm not going to judge. Do not do things that drain your will to live because cancer is already doing a fine job of that already.

But if I use the cancer card, then I have to tell people I have cancer and that's embarrassing.

Some people are 100% embarrassed they have cancer. First, if you are among these people, please immediately skip to

Chapter Eighteen: Cancer Isn't Your Fault. Also, re-read Chapter Five: Martyrs Die Alone. Second, check your own feelings about the people you know.

When you hear that someone has cancer do *you* say, "Ew, so gross—I bet they're gross odd weirdos and that's why they're sick."

Obviously, not.

Yet, plenty of people feel embarrassed that they got cancer, as if it somehow reflects badly on them.

It doesn't.

It feels gauche to play the Cancer Card.

Really? Since when is being honest crude? You're not making this shit up. You're not faking cancer. You are genuinely sick, and you will suffer a whole helluva lot with no one looking, so why not get out of bullshit that will impede your recovery?

Real friends will understand this.

Even frenemies will understand this.

The Cancer Card is so hard to counter because cancer cuts through politics and passive-aggressive pettiness. Cancer doesn't care how rich or poor you are, how famous you are, or how pretty or skinny you are. It blows up your life no matter who you are.

Everyone knows this. Everyone also knows they are not safe either. No one is safe as long as cancer exists.

So play that damn card.

Pep talk #15:

Hey there, people pleaser. Have you always had a hard time saying no? Well, then, it's your lucky day because now you have the perfect excuse to say no.

Say it early. Say it often. Shout it from the rooftops.

Noooooooooooooooooooooo!

You'll discover no one is mad at you at all. It's glorious. And so are you.

Do not feel guilty. Do not feel bad. You are saying no for the best reason of all: so you can fight another day.

Chapter Sixteen

Why Do I Still Have to Empty the Dishwasher and Attend Pointless Zoom Meetings? Responsibilities That Don't Magically Disappear

"Courage doesn't always roar. Sometimes courage is the little voice at the end of the day that says, 'I'll try again tomorrow.'"

—Mary Anne Radmacher

"Sometimes even to live is an act of courage."

—Seneca

As much as I believe the Cancer Card trumps all, it doesn't actually work when it comes to your mundane day-to-day responsibilities. Sometimes, you still have to do laundry, and we both know you won't be able to get out of *every* Zoom meeting for work.

You might feel resentful that life doesn't stop because you're waiting for your *billionth* biopsy result or your boss gets salty with you because you can't attend a meeting/convention/whatever because you've got an MRI scheduled. Your adolescent or twenty-something children or grandchildren don't miraculously have problem-free lives just because you're getting your weekly dose of chemo.

So, life goes on.

And that's infuriating. You're battling a fucking malignant demon, and Dan wants to know when you'll have those spreadsheets ready, per his last email? Just as soon as you start pulling your own weight around here, Dan. When will *that* happen?

You'll be expected to do more than fight cancer (though, be assured—that should always be your top priority right now).

When I was diagnosed with cancer, I'd just finished edits on a new novel, *The Takeover*, set to launch in four months.

For those of you not familiar with traditional publishing, publishers typically make their calendars SO far in advance. I'd held that publishing slot for more than a year. Many months before a book's release, they send out advanced copies to readers, trying to drum up interest and early reviews. You don't just easily "move" a book launch date, especially when all the marketing wheels are already in motion.

This was a difficult fact to explain to my oncologist when I told her about the book signings (some already scheduled!) and the book launch events planned.

"I'm sure you can just move the date," she'd said and shrugged.

That's not how these things work.

"Move the date?" my husband, PJ, said, aghast. "If you were a Ph.D. doctoral candidate, and you'd done work for years, and now you were going to defend your dissertation, do you just ask to *reschedule* for months later? No. You don't get to reschedule. You've got to do it now."

Have I mentioned how much I love my husband? He gets it.

He's seen me bust my ass making deadlines because they're not suggestions. People sometimes assume—completely wrongly—that romance writing isn't a serious profession. It's the most serious of professions. If I miss my deadline, if I back out of my contractual obligations, it's no different than if I were a real estate agent who failed to post a listing or a lawyer who simply chose not to file a brief because "life got in the way." Making a deadline can often mean the difference between making money and making no money at all. Also, if I don't fulfill my obligations, the publisher could, rightly, ask for their advance back.

Imagine if you showed up for work one day, and your boss was like, "Hey, you missed work last week. You owe us half the salary you already earned this year. Pay up."

Right. So, tell me again about how romance writing is an easy profession.

If I'd told the publisher to call off the launch date, it would've confused readers and reviewers alike. I would've lost the momentum the publisher (and I) had been building around the release date for many, many freakin' months. I would've disappointed readers, and in this media-blitzing, content-overload society, if I lost their attention, I might never gain it back. If I'd delayed the launch of my book eighteen months, I might have very well seen my sales halved.

And then all that hard work—of writing it, promoting it—would be for naught.

Deadlines are so important in publishing that I was once handed revisions and edits a mere day after I delivered my first baby in the hospital. My editor was rife with apologies, but could I just get them and finish the revisions in a month?

Yeah. Novelists—contract workers who can be cut for any time for any reason—get no "vacation days" or "maternity leave" or "sick leave" officially because they're not full-time workers; they're contract freelancers. They're disposable. Period.

Also, the tricky thing about promoting a book is that. . . well, you've got to show your face in public. At book signings and conferences and all over social media.

And I was about to have to start chemo, lose my hair, and still try to promote my book. It was kind of a nightmare. I've never been an overly vain person. I like to not look like an ogre, and I do worry a normal amount about walking around with spinach in my teeth, but I've never been so vain that my world revolved around what I looked like.

I felt like, of all people, I didn't really need this lesson in vanity. I didn't need to have to meet a bunch of new people while missing eyebrows and wearing scarves. Yet, it happened.

I *could* use the Cancer Card, but at the same time, this book was my baby. Did I want to abandon it now? Did I want to risk the work I'd put into it to all be for naught? No, I did not. This was one of those things I decided cancer simply wasn't going to take from me.

So, I penciled in my eyebrows and wore wigs and the N95 masks that my oncologist insisted I put on if I was going to be in a crowd. I went ahead and did all the book signings and the book conferences anyway. And while I hated not feeling my most beautiful self, I was also proud I hadn't given up. That I'd fought hard to get that book out into the world.

And in the end? That book—*The Takeover*? It hit the *USA Today* bestseller list.

Work and life won't stop, but sometimes that's a good thing.
You might want to throw a pity party for yourself because you've got all these things life requires you to do even while you're fighting cancer. You've got work obligations (maybe a couple of book readings and signings) and why? All you want to do is crawl into bed and watch trashy reality TV.

But there's an upside to being busy.

Being busy—working, taking care of your family, meeting obligations—gives you something to do other than fixate on cancer.

Your responsibilities might be a pain in the ass, but they're also wonderful at the same time.

If you're a lawyer, accountant, or kick-ass short order cook. . . if you're a teacher or a parent or a dogsitter. . .

whatever it is you do when you aren't battling cancer, you still ARE.

Isn't that amazing?

You're not simply a breast cancer patient. You're not helpless and sickly.

You've got a rich life. You play many roles, contribute to society in all kinds of amazing ways, and you will STILL do that, even when you're fighting cancer because you, my friend, are a badass.

Don't put down any of the labels that make you great. Don't shy away from the work and accomplishments that make you, *you*. When you're knee-deep in spreadsheets or management meetings, you're not thinking about death and chemo and whatever your cancer is doing, and that's good.

Embrace the work. Embrace the distraction.

Let's face it—we've been fighting for work-life balance all our lives and it's about to get a whole lot worse.

We may not have mastered the art of balancing work and life and family, but we've spent all our years desperately trying. Cancer is simply something else you'll be asked to manage, another plate to throw up on a stick as you balance the others: taking care of parents, working, networking, caring for children or pets, trying to squeeze in a moment of relaxation.

You've got plenty of practice at this. Now is the time to actually put all those skills you've spent a lifetime honing to work.

And it's also time to ditch all the bad habits because you literally can't afford them anymore. This isn't just some generic "stress" level you're talking about or "self-care," if and when you can squeeze it in. This is your LIFE we're talking about.

So, it's time to get crystal clear on what's important and what's not. But how?

The Five Ball Theory

In a 1991 Georgia Tech commencement speech by Coca-Cola CEO Brian Dyson, he urged the graduates to think of their lives as if they're juggling five balls: work, family, health, friends, and spirit. He says a ball like work is rubber. Drop it, and it'll bounce back. But there are other balls—like family, which are glass. Drop them and they'll break or crack.

It's our job to figure out which balls are glass and which are rubber.

And we also know that in life you have FAR more than five fucking balls in the air at any given time because we're not a billionaire CEO. There's the clean house ball, and the cooking ball, and the self-care ball. There's the taking care of pets ball, and the making sure you get all the birthday gifts in the mail in time ball, the volunteering at the school ball, the fixing the car ball, and the keeping up with the news ball.

There are a million fucking balls.

Spoiler: most of them are rubber.

But even with cancer, you're going to be expected to keep a lot of balls in the air. But also—many of them—might turn temporarily into rubber. Not forever, just temporarily.

I'll tell you what I mean.

The friendship ball. This is a ball you're supposed to cherish and protect, the one to keep from ever dropping on the ground.

But now is the time for your true friends to pitch in and help you—not the other way around. Right now, it's okay not to be available for gossip sessions (unless you want to be) and to say no to things you'd normally say yes to like dinners out (unless you want to go). You've invested a lot of time and effort in your friends over the years, and now, when you're sick, it's your turn to take some of that goodwill out of the bank.

So don't tie yourself into knots trying to get out to celebrate your friend's birthday if you've barely got enough energy to drag yourself out of bed.

Your friends—if they're true friends—will understand. They'll bring the party to you, or they'll celebrate with you later when you're feeling better.

Let's look at the spirituality ball. Well, maybe now you focus in on that ball, maybe it's a source of your strength—maybe you reconnect with your faith.

Or maybe you're too pissed off right now to do this.

That's okay, too.

You can play the Cancer Card with yourself, too. Don't forget. Get back to deep spiritual healing or reconnect with your best friend from high school later—when you've kicked cancer's ass.

Also, I hate to say this, but bad news doesn't stop just because you've got cancer.

If the universe were fair and perfect, then it would let you get cancer, and the bad news for the year—or fucking decade—would stop there.

But it doesn't.

Bad shit continues to happen that miraculously doesn't have anything to do with cancer. If you're like my Japanese grandmother, she'd tell you bad luck came in sevens (!).

For the release of *The Takeover*, I worked my butt off. I dragged myself bald to book events and conventions. I even did a book signing during chemotherapy with a mask after the bookstore had a COVID outbreak. I *showed up*.

And, as I mentioned before, that book became a bestseller.

And then, paradoxically, I got cut from my publisher.

During chemo.

The sales numbers weren't where they should be—even on a bestseller list (!!)—if you can believe it. Even hitting a list doesn't guarantee you a new contract these days. I hadn't met my numbers and now I was gone. It was a business decision, of course. Everyone I worked with felt terrible. Of course, they did. No one wants to fire someone in the middle of a cancer battle.

But it happens all the fucking time. Actually, in a survey conducted by BreastCancer.org, eighty-three percent of respondents said breast cancer affected their careers at least somewhat negatively. Fifty-one percent said "very to extremely negatively".[46] That's a whole lot. Let's face it: Bosses want to be understanding, but many of them, well, they simply aren't. That's the reality.

And it's hard to be your best self at work when you're fighting cancer. You might have to take a disability leave of absence. You may lose out on that next promotion. There are a million things that happen at work while you're at the cancer treatment center or recovering in the hospital.

Fight the battle in front of you.

The career ball is a glass ball. Or is it? Maybe it can be one of those glass-balls-that-are-temporarily-rubber-balls.

Because even if you drop it, it'll be okay. Fight cancer now, so you can live another day to fight for your career.

I've spent twenty-five years in publishing, and I've been cut from almost ALL of the big five publishers—and one, twice. This is just the nature of the business. It's cutthroat, I tell you. I've written forty books (and counting), and you've got to have nerves of steel for this business.

People who hear this think it's so awful, so horribly cold and terrible, but the thing is—getting fired during cancer did NOT hit me as hard as it would've if I'd been healthy.

I'd been getting such a shitty diet of terrible news (you don't need chemo, oh, wait you do need chemo! Also, chemo sucks ass! Get it and—you may shave years off your life, or

---

[46] Special Report: The Cost of Breast Cancer Care by Jen Uscher, BreastCancer.org.

don't get it and die next year! Maybe. We don't know. Wheeeeee!!!), that getting fired just didn't hit me as hard. Getting fired seemed small compared to *maybe dying*.

And I'd been in publishing for years. I'd been cut SO many times. And I'd come back. Again and again. Hell, I'm writing this book right now.

So, I knew I'd be back.

And frankly, it's hard to summon up shock and outrage when you're fighting cancer. Few things rise to that level of urgency.

Bad things will continue to happen, but you'll deal with them like the bad-ass warrior you are.

Pep talk #16:

Hey, Fighter. Life getting you down? Tired of having to juggle everything AND cancer, too? Wish the world would stop so you could get off this crazy ride? Don't.

All those responsibilities mean that people in your life need you. And isn't it good to be needed? To feel useful? I bet you want to feel a little less useful right now so you can go lie down and take a nap.

Remember that some things in life are rubber balls, and some are glass. It's okay to drop some things. And right now, there are more rubber balls in your life than ever.

They'll bounce up and be fine.

You have been juggling balls your whole life. You're an EX-PERT damn juggler, a Cirque Du Soleil-level circus performer. You know how to juggle.

Cancer is the biggest damn glass ball of all, but you can toss it and keep it in the air with all the rest.

You're an amazing miracle of a performer. You always have been. You can do this. I know you can.

Chapter Seventeen

Cut Out Toxic People—You Can Only Deal with One Malignant Asshole at a Time, and Right Now That's Cancer

"Surround yourself only with people who are going to lift you higher."

—Oprah Winfrey

Cancer will help you realize there's a lot of bullshit in your life.

It's a valuable lesson that can only come when you're facing an acute crisis. Take the 2020 COVID Pandemic. Facing potential death during a worldwide shutdown left many people realizing—hey, my shitty job with my shittier boss isn't worth my high blood pressure—and many people quit. So many people quit that they called it The Great Resignation.[47]

Difficult times bring clarity for many.

This is true of cancer.

Cancer helps you focus on what's important and what's bullshit in your life. The things you would've sworn were EVERYTHING last week—that promotion, your grandkid getting playing time on his basketball team, your neighbor finally mowing his lawn—all of that will fade into the background, becoming small and inconsequential. In the hierarchy of needs, we have to first *be alive* to get to cherry-pick everything else.

---

[47] Hubert Janicki, "How the COVID-19 Pandemic Prompted More People to Change Jobs," Census.gov, May 13, 2024.

You might discover that you've been tolerating people in your life that are toxic.

When you're well, you can deal with a whole lot of bullshit. When you're healthy, you can tolerate all kinds of toxicity from a whole bunch of people. It can come in all forms: a narcissistic spouse, a passive-aggressive parent, a backstabbing friend who spreads gossip about you, a scheming coworker who regularly takes credit for your work or sets you up to fail. You all know who I mean.

If you're lucky, when cancer explodes into your life, you've already dealt with toxicity, and you live a life as toxic-free as possible.

Before I met and married my husband, PJ, I found myself in an emotionally abusive relationship. This person was jealous of everything I'd accomplished—of being a published author, working from home, having good friends, being a self-sufficient single mom. He told me he was there to support and protect me, except what he did instead was chip away at my self-esteem, gaslight me, separate me from friends and family, use me for my money (after pushing for me to buy a house that we could all live in, only to move in and then never, actually, pay a dime towards the mortgage or anything else), and then eventually he sent out a whole bunch of texts one drunken night looking to hook up with a woman he'd sworn to me he never had any interest in.

Right.

But love is blind, you know? It was hard to see the truth when I was so busy desperately ignoring all the red flags.

Emotional abuse (like any abuse) doesn't happen over-night. I was a frog in a pot of water, slowly being brought to a boil. I always counted myself as a thoughtful person. One day I bought the wrong brand of cheese from the grocery store, except I am 100% sure we'd had that cheese many times before. He ranted and raved about how I was thoughtless and cruel, how I didn't even know him because, if I *did*, I would've known he hated that fucking brand of cheese.

All I could do was apologize—profusely—even though part of me knew I was being gaslit. Part of me *knew* I'd bought that cheese before. Not every grocery trip, but enough times. Hell, it was hard to *avoid* that brand of cheese. It's everywhere! And this story he was telling me about how he hated that brand, well, it was new to me. Since when? And since when do people go bonkers over a cheese brand? Is there that much difference between Kraft and Boar's Head? Apparently, there is.

Also, he talked a lot about wanting to take care of me, except when I needed something, really needed something, he was never there. When I wanted my oldest and dearest friend to come visit, he'd pick apart everything she said or did, making it an insult to him (How DARE she ask for her glass of wine to be refilled in *that* completely normal tone? He's not her servant, and by the way, she's never allowed in *his* house that he never paid for and isn't on the mortgage because she dared to disrespect him by not saying please).

Then, of course, any one of my friends, or my mother, expressing how they worried about the way he treated me, well, *they* were the problem, weren't they? *They* didn't have my true interests at heart, not like he did. They were the problem, not him, and if *I* loved him, I'd show my loyalty and cut them out of my life.

Here's a spoiler alert, ladies, if your partner is asking you to prove your love to them all the time by cutting out people who really do love you, then your spouse does not love you. If they're constantly telling you that you are a terrible, inconsiderate person for forgetting things you are 100% sure you didn't forget, that's not love.

That's abuse.

Love does not blame. Love is not jealous. Love is not psychotically obsessed with certain brands of cheese.

When I'd discovered he'd been trying to hook up with another woman behind my back, he tried to gaslight me about those too. He never sent any text messages, he said. Someone else must have snuck into his room at night and sent them from his phone. Or his friend did it as a prank. I shouldn't believe what's right in front of my face. That was truly the last straw. At that point, I realized he'd withdrawn all the good will in the bank by ranting about my friends and family and, of course, cheese. There was nothing there for him to draw on. His balance was empty.

So, I cut ties. It was horrible, heartbreaking, and scary. I was in a bigger house that I'd wanted or thought I could afford, because I thought we'd be getting married and splitting the mortgage. I had no idea how I'd cover the expenses. I'd moved away from close friends so I could afford more space, and now I felt marooned on a suburban island, not sure what I should do next.

That was a bleak time.

But an important time.

After I found some extra freelance work, and picked myself up and dusted myself off, I began dating again.

And... amazingly, I found my fantastic husband, PJ. He lived closer to my new place than my old, and, honestly, if I'd never moved, I would've been out of the "geographically desirable" range, and I probably would never have connected with him because it would've been too hard to get together.

I don't know if you believe in fate, but I believe that the universe does try to put us on the right path, sometimes. It engineers events to happen just at the right time for the right reasons. Like me logging on to my ex's Apple computer to Google something after a reboot and seeing the texts he thought he deleted right there on the damn screen.

This isn't ALWAYS the case. I'm not saying this about cancer. I don't think it can really come at the right time, and there's never a right reason.

But I met PJ, my soulmate, my PERSON, seven years before I was diagnosed with breast cancer. And PJ has been my ROCK through this whole treatment.

I think back and wonder sometimes what would've happened if I'd been in my previous relationship, and I know it would've been awful. I spent so much time during my treatment, grateful, that I wasn't with him. Grateful that I wasn't battling a toxic emotional abuser at the same time as cancer.

If you're dealing with a toxic person, now is the time to cut ties.

I was so grateful not to be in that emotionally abusive relationship anymore, but that didn't mean I was completely free from all toxic people. They come in all forms—from the very minorly toxic to the completely noxious. As you focus on your own battle, you seriously cannot afford to let people drain your energy.

You need it. You need all of it.

So, in case you've never given yourself permission to avoid people who make your teeth hurt, I'm officially giving you permission to let these people go.

Hopefully, the toxic person is not front and center. Hopefully, the toxicity is on the outskirts. You do not owe anything to that old friend from college who keeps one-upping you in all the social media posts. You don't have to go to your friend's coworker's birthday party, where you only know one person, and you don't even like that person that much.

You don't have to tolerate a brother-in-law who mansplains YOUR OWN industry to you when he has zero knowledge of it, and never even graduated from college.

You don't need anyone draining your inner battery because cancer will do that every single day. You'll need all your energy to fight cancer, and you have none left over for anybody else's bullshit.

If a toxic person is close to you, then now is the time to reconsider whether this is someone you really do want to spend the rest of your life with. Trust me when I tell you, it will become abundantly clear if this person does not give a shit about you. They will not put you first. They will not be the support you need. They will think only of themselves.

They might even cheat when you're at your absolute sickest and then blame you for it because that's what toxic people do. They are selfish to their core, and this will be on display, front and center, when you need their help the most in this most dire of battles.

Set boundaries and defend them.

Cutting out toxic people doesn't necessarily mean never talking to them or having a big blow up with them in your life (though it CAN mean that—and the more toxic they are, the more I encourage you to cut them completely out).

But having cancer gives you the perfect excuse (remember that Cancer Card?) to set boundaries now and decide who you want to see more of in your life and who you'd like to see less.

Take this time to weed out people who drain you.

If you've never set boundaries before, hang on, honey. Shit's about to get real.

Some of you may be very good at setting boundaries. You may have already spent most of your adult life honing the skill. For others of you, this might be the very first time you told your spouse that *No, you won't be going over to his ex-wife's house this*

Thanksgiving and Christmas Eve for the kids who are now 30 and 33, respectively.

If you're brand new to setting boundaries with other people, know that they won't make it easy for you. Some of them will guilt you and bully you and gaslight you.[48] But stick to your guns, anyway.

How can you learn to say no?

It all starts with *knowing your worth*. You are valuable. Your time is valuable. You are trying to kick cancer's ass and that's IMPORTANT. Toxic people will try to convince you that they're more important than you are. They'll probably even want you to think about how hard it is for them dealing with your cancer.

DO NOT APOLOGIZE for what you need. You can say no, and you do NOT have to be sorry about it.

And right now, you're going to have to speak clearly about what you want and stick to it. If you've never properly articulated your wants and needs in your family or circle of friends, then it's going to feel weird and awkward the first few times you do it. But it's just a muscle you haven't used very often. The more you use it, the easier it will become.

And, trust me, it's worth it.

Set those boundaries early and defend them with all you've got.

And then—an amazing thing will happen. You will start to feel great. Like, really, fantastically great. You're asking for what you want. You're getting what you need. Your battery—instead of being drained—will be full and recharged and ready for the battle ahead.

---

[48] Jason Whiting Ph.D., "How to Stand Up for Yourself With Toxic People," *Psychology Today*, November 20, 2020.

Pep talk #17:

Hey, Warrior. You can't be in the trenches with backstabbers and traitors.

You can't go to war with people who don't have your back. Time to let the shitty and toxic people go. They'll just fuck things up on the battlefield. They will cut and run every damn time.

Don't feel bad about cutting them out of your life. You were never going to be good enough for them anyway because they're not good enough for themselves.

That's why they're toxic and you're not. It's better to be alone than to be with people who will drag you down.

Gallop onto the battlefield with sword on fire, confident your army is within you.

Chapter Eighteen

Cancer Isn't Your Fault.
Don't Waste Time on Regret.

"You, yourself, as much as anyone else in the entire universe, deserve your love and affection."

—Buddha

I was three and a half months late getting my annual mammogram in August 2023. I'd gone to my ob-gyn annual exam (also about three or four months late—because. . . life). I'd been in deadline hell, getting my book to my editor and working on revisions, and also, by the way, pitching in to help my husband launch his new logistics franchise, all while being a mom and stepmom and dog mom—whose responsibilities never, ever ended.

"Have you gotten your mammogram this year?" my ob-gyn asked, as she did every year.

I thought about it a minute. Wait. . . didn't I have one scheduled two months ago? Yeah, I did. I had to cancel for a reason I couldn't quite remember—maybe one of the kids was home sick, or maybe I had a work call, or some reason I'd canceled. And—huh—I'd never rescheduled now that I thought about it.

"No," I said. "But it's on my list." It wasn't until right then—but, oh well. These kinds of wellness exams and tests always felt like rubber balls. The kind you could drop. I was always juggling so many glass balls that, well, the rubber ones always got dropped. Sometimes more than once.

"You really should get that done," she scolded me.

Fine, I thought. *I will.*

And I did, pretty much, get my mammogram every year since I was forty-five (though new guidelines suggest people start at 40). It might be more like every fifteen to seventeen months or so, but I GOT it on a regular basis for years.

But I also started to do the calculations and realized our COBRA was running out at the end of that same month—September—so I might as well get my money's worth out of the overly expensive insurance before we got spun out into a big old question mark.

Some of you will be lucky enough to never know a single day in your life without medical coverage. The rest of us deal with this ebb and flow of whether or not we're covered *all the time.* Health insurance is less of a solid, dependable staple and more of a delicacy or treat—something we get when we can afford it, or when it's available or in season, like a rare fruit.

My husband and I talked about probably just going without insurance for the last quarter of the year, maybe just head to the Marketplace (Affordable Care Act) which I'd been on and off for most of the last fifteen years.

We were debating, of course, though we only had a few weeks to decide, but it didn't seem that urgent. It never does. Health insurance is one of those expenses that feels distant and unimportant but can become vital overnight.

I spent weeks beating myself up.

I had breast cancer and I'd waited *three and a half months.* What would I do with myself if those three and a half months meant the difference between Stage 1 and Stage 2?

Oh, I berated myself for putting it off, for thinking it was a rubber ball, when clearly health was a damn glass ball, and now I'd dropped it and broken it.

And let's not even get into the point where I started spinning out about losing health insurance. Why had I left the *diagnostic* test to the end when I was almost out of insurance?

Because I was confident it would be negative, and just one more box to check off.

"One month or two, doesn't make that much difference."

My breast surgeon, the blunt, tell-it-like-it-is, pull-no-punches surgeon was explaining that my delayed mammogram probably, in the end, wouldn't really affect the outcome. "Now, if you'd waited a year? Then we'd have serious problems."

I clung to her words, stupidly relieved that I could tell myself *I'd gotten the mammogram* in time, and that I hadn't dropped the glass ball after all.

"And you've gotten mammograms every year so we know what's changed," the surgeon told me. And I patted myself on the back. I'd gotten them (mostly!) regularly! I'd been responsible!

But let's face it: you can't change what's happened in the past. You don't know what the future holds, so you can only face the present.

Even if I had put off that mammogram for a year, I'd still need to deal with what's right in front of me. And, honestly, if my ob-gyn hadn't reminded me about the mammogram, maybe I would've gone a whole other year—or at least until the next October—and saw breast cancer awareness ribbon banners on my social media, before remembering that *Oh, yeah, I've got to schedule one of those!*

So, the fact is, I had to let go of the guilt and stop kicking myself, and so do you. Whatever happened in the past, however late your mammogram was, whatever you ate or didn't eat, or whatever deodorant you used. . . it really doesn't matter now.

Now you're facing what you're facing, and it's about squaring your shoulders, and ditching the woulda, coulda, shoulda. Those times are gone.

Fuck it. Even if you shot-gunned weed killer every night of your life and smoked three packs a day, this cancer isn't your fault. Stop looking for reasons to take blame for it, and don't allow anyone to saddle you with blame for it. Cancer is a messy bitch, and you did not invite her into your life.

You have to deal with HER consequences right now, and you do not have time to beat yourself up about that mammogram you missed.

What you *can* do is make sure there are NO woulda, coulda, shouldas in the future. That means making decisions now you believe will minimize your chance of regret later.

Nobody asks for cancer.

Even if you might have been careless about your own health, you didn't ask for cancer. No one does. You could've done every single risky behavior—early and often—but you're still not asking for cancer. We're human. Maybe we drink or eat too much, sometimes, and maybe we don't eat heathy foods or move around as much as we should. Because we think we're invincible and it won't happen to us.

It's not your fault you got cancer.

Some people truly believe they can *give* themselves cancer. But this is not how cancer works.[49]

Full stop.

It's CANCER's fault you got cancer.

She's a messy bitch—we already agreed. I cannot say this enough: cancer will try to distract you with problems that

---

[49] "Effect of Attitudes and Feelings on Cancer," American Cancer Society, 2023.

aren't problems. It will divert your energy to things that don't help you fight it.

Spending a lot of time kicking yourself for anything that happened in the past doesn't help you focus on the now.

She's the one you SHOULD be mad at, not yourself, okay? Be angry. Be furious—AT CANCER.

Okay? Okay.

Blaming ourselves is a form of emotional abuse.[50]

The blame game isn't harmless. The negative playlist in our heads isn't harmless, either. Psychologists will tell you that self-blame is a form of emotional abuse. Focusing on self-blame doesn't help us address the problem in front of us, it just make us feel less competent to handle it.

Spoiler alert: we are all just messy humans. We make mistakes. We don't mean to make mistakes but we make them.

Michael Formica wrote in *Psychology Today*: "The key to self-acceptance—the lynchpin in the system of becoming a whole human—is recognizing that we are perfect just the way we are and that perfection is stunningly imperfect. In fact, it's a mess—an absolutely beautiful disaster. It's, well, human."

First, we should really embrace the idea that we're not perfect and that's okay, and then, we must move towards responsibility.

Responsibility is different from blame. Blame assigns shame and negative feelings to a condition. Blame makes us feel shameful and unworthy. Responsibility is simply admitting to a mistake.

I'll show you the difference between blame and responsibility.

---

[50] Michael J. Formica EdM, NCC, LPC, "Self-Blame: The Ultimate Emotional Abuse," *Psychology Today*, April 19, 2013.

You're out to brunch with your girlfriends, and you each get a separate check. You initially miscalculate the tip on the bill, but you look at your friend's receipt and you see your mistake. If you're in the blame game you tell yourself: *God, you're such a moron. You never get math right. You can't do anything right. You're an idiot.*

Taking responsibility means you say, *Oops. I made a mistake. I'll just cross this amount out, put the new one in, and problem solved.*

See the difference? One is super negative and mean, and the other is all about acknowledgment, correcting the mistake, and moving on.

Pause the playlist of negative self-talk in your head.

Getting away from blame is difficult because most of us have a mixtape of negative thoughts in our brains. They're put there by a society that doesn't value us, by our parents who meant well, but perhaps were overly critical of us, or by our friends or lovers or teachers or classmates, and finally, by ourselves because we just love to pile on.

I'm sure you know this playlist already.

You shouldn't have said that. You always say the wrong thing.

You should never try that. You're going to fail, and people are going to laugh at you.

Just be quiet. Don't start trouble. You always want to start something.

You don't deserve that promotion. You're an impostor and everyone will find out soon enough.

You're going to try to write a book? Please. That's way too hard for you. And no one will want to read it, anyway. Don't even try.

That negative self-talk in our brains often goes on a loop, in the background, and we don't even know it's there.

There's an amazing movie about this. It's called *Violet*, directed by Justine Bateman. In the movie, Olivia Munn plays Violet—a successful film executive with a never-ending loop of negative thoughts in her brain (voiced by Justin Theroux), which second-guesses every single decision she makes. Think about the worst peanut gallery on earth. When you watch it, as an audience member, you KNOW that voice is lying. That voice is telling *Olivia Munn* she's ugly? What is that voice smoking?! But you also recognize that voice. It's the voice in all our heads telling us we're not good enough.

"Years ago, I made a lot of fear-based decisions, and so when I got to the other side of that, I knew that I had a lot of time stolen from me where I hadn't been myself," Bateman said during the screening of the film at Northwestern's Chicago campus in 2022. "I wanted to exact revenge, so I made this film so that someone else could watch it and realize the voice, the negative voice, was lying, and the opposite was probably true."[51]

We all have negative self-talk in our heads, and it's usually put there by a parent, a friend, or a teacher. Someone who made a big impression on us when we were growing up.

"The musings of your inner critic may sound a lot like a critical parent or friend from your past. It can follow the path of typical cognitive distortions: catastrophizing, blaming, and the like," said Elizabeth Scott, Ph.D., an author and educator who promotes the value of positive thinking.

Scott said negative self-talk typically falls into five camps:

- Negativity disguised by practicality ("Learning to ski? That's too dangerous.")
- Mean ("I always mess everything up.")

---

[51] Cara Lockwood, "Filmmaker Justine Bateman Discusses 'Violet' as Part of Pritzker Pucker Studio Lab Programming," Northwestern School of Communication, February 9, 2022.

- Hopeless ("Nothing good happens for me because I don't deserve it.")
- Apathetic ("Why try? I'm just going to fail.")
- Defeated—usually before we even try to do something ("Why even try to run a marathon? It's way too hard and I won't be able to do it.")[52]

That inner negative critic will have a field day with a breast cancer diagnosis. Now, we have a whole lot more to blame ourselves for and, boy, are we gluttons for punishment.

Here's where things get real. You've been beating yourself up with a mean playlist in your head for years, but now, those thoughts aren't just stealing away your calm and your happiness; they might be actually taking your life. The problem with self-blame is that it leads to worse outcomes. Negative self-talk is linked to greater stress, lower lifespans, poor cardiac health, and even a greater risk of dying from cancer. Positive self-talk can be a superpower, to help you recover from infections, beat cancer, and just be happier.[53]

So how do we stop the loop of negativity in our brains?

It doesn't happen overnight. But the first step is to recognize the playlist when it starts to play. When the negative thoughts begin to churn in the back of your mind, stop and listen. Call out that thought. Is this something you'd say to your own child? Your best friend? Someone you manage in your office? Then, why are you saying it to yourself?

Next step? Separate your inner critic from yourself. Give her a name. Call her Karen. Call her Debbie Downer. Or

---

[52] Elizabeth Scott, Ph.D, "The Toxic Effects of Negative Self-Talk," *Very Well Mind*, November 22, 2023.

[53] "Positive thinking: Stop negative self-talk to reduce stress," *The Mayo Clinic*, November 21, 2023.

Negative Nancy. Call her whatever you want. But then when a thought like, "*I can't do chemo. It's too hard*," pops into your head, you know that's Karen talking.

Give Karen or the playlist a limit on how long you'll let the negative thoughts run. Don't listen to Karen's playlist all day, every day. Tell yourself you'll only allow her to play her favorite hits for a certain amount of time a day or only on a certain subject. Cancer treatment is off-limits. Let her rail about how you fold towels, sure, but how you recover from surgery? Nope. She doesn't get to talk about that. And if she does want to talk about it? Demand she change her negativity to neutrality. "I can't do radiation" becomes "Radiation is hard." See how different that is? You acknowledge radiation is a rough road, but you don't tell yourself it's impossible at the same time. You don't tell yourself you're going to fail before you even try.

Go a step further than this. Argue with your inner critic. Challenge her. Does that bitch even know what she's talking about? My bet is no. She just yaps all day in your brain, talking all kinds of smack, but has NOTHING to back it up with. She has zero receipts. Once you start actively challenging that negative loop in your brain, you might be surprised to discover there's no there, there. The more you challenge those thoughts, the more they become silly and ridiculous and will have less of a hold on you.

These thoughts only have power because, like Violet in the movie, we just let them run without challenging them. Once we challenge them, once we call them out, we take away their power.

Don't forget to give yourself the kudos you deserve.
Leading up to my double mastectomy, I had a whole bunch of thoughts in my brain. Most of them were along the lines of: *Maybe we can still sneak on a flight to Barbados! I hear it's lovely this time of year! Let's run away!* So—that's the fear talking,

obviously. Fear always wants to give you the easy way out (which, by the way, is never the easy way out. It's always harder.).

But I also had some negative self-talk in my brain because—of course, I did—and those thoughts went like, *This will be painful and you won't be able to handle it. You're going to embarrass yourself. The doctors and nurses will be disappointed in you and talk about what a terrible patient you are. You're going to cry and blubber and make a scene, and then everyone will know you're weak. Maybe you'll get addicted to pain meds. After this surgery, you'll look like a freak no one can love. Everyone will reject you.*

I mean, my inner critic is a real bitch, okay?

I'd fought these thoughts for weeks before my surgery. I fought them by hitting the treadmill and pumping weights. Every day, my muscles were sore. I handled that pain, so I told myself I'd be able to handle the surgical pain, too. I tried to eat right. I talked to my counselor, so I felt my emotions in real time and didn't stuff them down. I talked about my fears aloud—about being a freak, about feeling unlovable. When I dragged these horrible thoughts out into the light, they became less scary. Because scary things are always less scary in the bright light of day, and because I realized how ridiculous they sounded.

They were ridiculous because none of them were true.

After the surgery, I wasn't weak. I was strong. Stronger than I even gave myself credit for being. I'd faced my fear. I punched my fear in the face. My husband didn't reject me. He praised my courage and strength. My kids loved me even more, grateful I was still here and I'd survived. The pain was manageable. It didn't control me. I didn't get addicted to painkillers because I didn't take that many. The doctors and nurses praised my positive attitude because I cracked jokes with them before going into surgery. They told me I was a stellar patient.

It just proved those negative thoughts before the surgery were lies.

Spoiler alert: those negative thoughts are ALWAYS lies.

So after the surgery, during a quiet time one morning, I congratulated myself. I told myself, "You did a good job, kid." It was the same no-nonsense gruff way my dad would've patted me on the back when I was growing up.

And I instantly started crying.

I bawled because I knew this was the truth. I DID a good job. I powered through. I met every challenge. I didn't embarrass myself or anyone else. I ROSE to that fucking occasion. I soldiered through a traumatic surgery with grace. I surprised MYSELF by how well I did.

I also was crying because I realized *how rare it was in my life that I really, truly gave myself genuine praise.*

I cheer on my friends and family and work colleagues all the time. But I NEVER did that for myself. The best I could hope for when I achieved a goal (published my first book, got my first movie, hit the USA Today bestseller list) was typically a backhanded compliment. *Sure, you got one book published, but maybe it's a fluke, and you're a fake because your second book didn't sell. Oh, that movie they made out of your book? Yeah. I mean good for you but it's not a major motion picture, is it? What was that? A little cable movie? Bet no one will watch it, either. Oh? You hit the* USA Today *list? I mean, good for you, I guess? It's not the* New York Times *bestseller list, but I mean, celebrate if you want.*

Seriously, the negative self-talk? Bad. Real bad. It didn't stop when I accomplished things. *Oh, you gave birth? Great. But you don't know how to get that baby to stop crying, and the baby won't latch, so you're a failure.*

Sound familiar? I bet it does.

But this time, with the surgery? I didn't allow negative thoughts. I didn't allow back-handed compliments. My body was facing a traumatic surgery, we came out of it with flying colors, and I gave myself genuine praise. It was genuine because I'd been scared AF that we wouldn't make it through. But we did. There was no, *Good for you, but. . .* There was simple praise.

I encourage you to do this for yourself. Cheer for *you*, honestly and loudly and often, especially in this fight for your life. And you'll discover something amazing. When you start cheering for yourself, when you give yourself honest kudos, you'll start to be more confident. You'll *know* in your bones you are capable, amazing, and awesome because it's the truth. You'll turn down the volume on that negativity playlist, and, hell, you might even mute it.

As you pass each challenge: crushing the surgery recovery, keeping your head high during chemo, gritting your teeth during radiation—you'll put another notch in your belt. The negative playlist can't take that from you. It can't argue with facts.

You ARE worthy.

You ARE amazing.

Pep talk #18:

Hey there, Fighter.

It's time to turn down the negative playlist in your head. Those tunes have been feeding you a pack of lies. Your inner critic is writing checks her ass can't cash. So, mute it.

You are a badass.

You are loveable.

You are capable and amazing and awesome.

You deserve to fucking LIVE.

You deserve love, and happiness and GOOD HEALTH.

Trust in yourself. You CAN do this. You will make it to the other side.

Chapter Nineteen

You Don't Have to Be a Gazelle.
It's Okay to Be a Bull in a China Shop.

"When you come to the end of your rope, tie a knot and hang on."

—Franklin D. Roosevelt

When I was first diagnosed, some people in my life really felt that the only way through cancer—the only way through the fight—was to be as joyful and positive as possible. Some people really cling to this idea that we've got to be joyful warriors (and you can be), but I'm also here to tell you that you can be salty and sarcastic, too. If you're a super upbeat person, sure, you can binge on those frilly sayings in the home décor section of *Home Goods*.

You can *live, laugh, love* to your heart's content. (Though, let's be real, you can't *live, laugh, love* all the time. Sometimes people *die, cry, hate* or *kill, curse, spite*. I mean, we're only human.) I had an acquaintance who plastered her entire home—every available surface—with such scripted uplifting little messages. She hated cursing and never wanted to acknowledge that bad things often happened to good people. She believed wholly in the power of manifestation, so in mind, if a single doubt or negative thought ever crept into her brain, she'd be dooming herself to abject failure.

She lived in a little bubble of positivity, which is, I repeat, totally FINE. I mean, I was kind of jealous because, if you haven't figured it out by now, I can be a bit. . . salty.

Now, after I announced my cancer, I tried to post funny videos online. Why? Because I was trying to stay fucking sane, and again—have we talked about how cancer and death have zero sense of humor? They are way too serious. Laughing at them felt sooooo good.

One of the videos I posted was how I felt about cancer, and I used a clip of Robert DeNiro as Al Capone in *The Untouchables*, where he's so mad at Elliot Ness for investigating him, he demands his lackeys to get him. "I want him dead," Al Capone rants. "I want his family dead. I want his house burned to the ground. I want to go there in the middle of the night and piss on his ashes."

My bubbly friend was so concerned when she saw this. "You have to be careful!" she cautioned me. "You've got to have a positive attitude!!"

So, I want to be crystal clear right now: you can want to murder cancer in the most gruesome ways possible and STILL have a positive attitude. You can go around ranting in your head, "I hope cancer *gets* cancer and fucking dies" and still have a positive attitude. You can want to destroy everything that cancer ever cared about, scorch every single safe haven until she has none, and still feel grateful to be alive.

Dig into your own personal Al Capone energy.

Because here's what I discovered: being angry was fine. It came with the territory. It happened all on its own. You don't always have to be a graceful ballerina. You can be a cursing brawler, too.

We often set impossible standards for ourselves. We're supposed to never fail, never complain, never stop smiling, and—God forbid—never fucking age. But sometimes life throws you some pretty nasty curveballs, and it's okay to be mad, to NOT be beautiful, not to have all the answers. During your cancer treatment, you'll not only learn some pretty tough lessons about your body, but you'll learn a lot about who you are.

I also want you to give yourself a fucking break.

You don't have to do everything right this time. You're fighting for your life. You will snap someone's head off. Someone might even call you difficult.

That's okay.

We don't have to be a fucking gazelle or an Instagram model during the fight of our lives. We just have to show up. Do you fear you don't have it in you to fight?

Let me remind you this isn't the first time in your life you've faced adversity.

If you've lived this long and managed never to have a setback, then I want to know your secret!

We've all had setbacks. Heartaches. Maybe even a divorce. Maybe we've been laid off or passed over for a promotion. Maybe we had parents who set expectations for us too damn high, or maybe we set expectations for the people who are supposed to love us too damn low.

Life comes with disappointments and setbacks, times when you had to find a deeper resolve to pick yourself up and keep going, even when you weren't sure about the destination anymore.

You've been through tough times before.

I want you to think about the last time life kicked you in the teeth. The time before cancer. Was it a divorce? An accident? Losing your job?

Life, no doubt, delivered some serious curveballs to you in the past.

You're still here. You're still here despite all that. And cancer will just be one more setback that helps you be more resilient, more adaptable, and strong as fuck.

Sometimes You Have to Adult Yourself

"So, it sounds to me like you just don't want to do this," my counselor tells me at her home office. I'm sitting on her leather couch, and I'm complaining about all the side effects of surgery, and how the doctors still don't know for sure if I'll need chemotherapy, and I'm just basically ranting.

"No, I don't," I said.

"You didn't ask for this," she points out.

"No, I didn't."

"You *can* do it. You *can* get through it. You just don't want to."

"Right." I mean I *guess I* can.

My counselor stomps her foot on the ground like a toddler. "I don't want to. You're like a toddler at the grocery store."

"Yes!" It's true. "I'm throwing a tantrum."

"And that's okay. It's okay not to want to do this. This is Plan B. Plan A was never to get cancer. This is Plan B."

"Right." God, did I never expect for this fucking Plan B. I never thought I'd be here.

"You *can* do it. You just don't want to."

I nod. The tears start flowing. I don't want to do this. I just don't. I'm supposed to get *happy* about getting a double mastectomy? I'm supposed to be relieved that they can treat this by slicing off chunks of me?

"You've been through tougher things than this. Emotional things. Things you didn't want to do."

Divorce. Telling my parents my marriage failed and it was my fault. That was far worse than this. I didn't even get pity then.

"You've given birth to two babies. That was real pain."

I nod. It was.

"You gave birth the first time and then you went back and had another."

It sounds insane now, but it's true. Not only did I have twenty hours of labor and gave birth to a nearly nine-pound baby (and I was just five foot one), but then I had a pelvic separation right after the birth and couldn't walk without the help of a walker for a full month. And then I had a second baby!

"You had the worst pain of your life and *then* you took care of a crying baby."

"And bleeding nipples!" I point out.

"Yes, sure! So, see? You *can* do this. You *will* do this. You'll beat this. You know why?"

"Why?" I almost don't want to know why.

"Because you have to."

She's right.

"You don't have a choice."

She's so right.

I may not have asked for this. I may not want this. This might be the worst Plan B of all time. But I'm here now. And there's only one way out. And that's straight through.

"You're strong. This will make you stronger. Listen, weak people? Truly weak people? They don't come to me. They don't sit there on that couch."

I nod.

"Strong people come to me. Strong people get stronger—in here."

The best weapon you have against cancer is your mind.
This sounds trite and stupid, I know.

But it's the truth.

The best weapon you have is your mind. Remember that negative playlist in your head? Can you mute it?

Are you strong? Are you a warrior? Are you ready to kick ass?

Or are you weak? Are you a victim? Do you not have any control over your life?

The way you go into surgery or treatment will be everything. And here's the best part: cancer doesn't get to decide your attitude. YOU decide. This is up to YOU.

But you're not strong enough, you tell me.

You're stronger than you know.

Why?

Because you have to be.

But you fear pain.

Who doesn't? Pain sucks! Nobody stands in line at Six Flags to get punched in the face. Pain is awful. We all hate it.

But you'll get through it.

Because you have to.

The fear feels like a tsunami wave meant to drown you in anxiety.

Fear sucks. Fear is the boogie man under the bed. Fear is worrying about whether this will bankrupt you. But the only way to deal with fear is to look it straight in the eye.

I see you, fear.

I see you.

You'll deal with the fear.

Because you have to.

Being strong doesn't mean you don't cry. Hell, it might mean you cry all the damn time.

Kicking ass doesn't mean that you do it gracefully with charm and a joke. It means that you keep on going. Nobody asked you to be a gazelle through the china shop. You're a goddamn bull. You might smash the gravy bowl, but you'll get through.

You will.

Because you have to.

I know what you saying right now because I've said it. I'm not a fighter. I'm not a warrior. I'm a suburban working mom who frets about how to graciously get out of helping with the bake sale. I'm a damn pacifist. I avoid conflict like the plague and would much rather curl up with a glass of wine and watch true crime or reality TV than ever, EVER bring up a disagreement with a friend.

But you've got a choice now.

You can be a victim. Or you can be a survivor.

Listen, I'll be a hundred percent honest with you: you'll get through the surgery, or the chemo, or the whatever, probably either way.

You'll either live feeling like a put-out victim.

Or you'll live feeling like a kick-ass warrior.

You can live either way.

But living as a victim will be more painful. It will be harder. There will be more fear. It's just the truth.

If you let cancer—or, really, anything in life – tell you how you're going to feel and how you're going to live, then what kind of life is that at all?

It's someone else's life because you're not living it. You're not in control.

This is YOUR life.

Not cancer's.

Cancer doesn't get to decide.

The treatments don't get to decide.

YOU get to decide.

Take power back when you can.

Pain for Gain

"When I gave birth to my son," my counselor tells me, "I told myself it was pain for gain. I was going through that to get a beautiful baby. So, for you, do the same now. Focus on pain for gain. Focus on the prize."

Getting healthy. Taking back my life. Focus on the living and thriving, less on the literal surviving.

"You've got to keep your eye on the prize," my counselor tells me. "Pain for gain."

When you give yourself permission to go messy, you might find you're a gazelle after all.

Early on in this process, I let myself off the hook for being perfect. I told myself I'd get a medal for getting through, even if I yelled and screamed all the way to the end. But you know what? I didn't yell and scream (all that much). I made it far more gracefully than I ever thought I would.

If you tell yourself early and often that you don't have to be perfect, you just might find, at the end of all of this, you've handled it all with dignity. Do you know why? When you show yourself grace and give yourself space to be human, you allow yourself the runway to be fucking amazing.

Constantly criticizing or second-guessing yourself makes you feel small and terrible, and people who feel small and terrible often lash out and do bad things. Hurt people hurt people.

You are doing all the hard work. You are facing your fear. You are putting one foot in front of the other. You are doing the hard work of being mentally healthy to fight this battle, and you are giving yourself permission to mess up—because we all mess up. And what comes from that is something beautiful and amazing. It's your transformation into a kick-ass warrior, someone I'd be proud to stand shoulder-to-shoulder with any day of the week.

Pep talk #19:

Hey, Gladiator. War is hard and it's ugly, and nobody expects you to do a pirouette while you're smashing cancer's face in. You don't have to do this like a graceful ballerina with your make-up perfect and never breaking a sweat. You can clomp awkwardly and break things.

The whole point is that you get to the other side. Whether you skip there or you crawl on your hands and knees, the point is to get there.

And you will, gladiator.

You are a giant slayer.

Chapter Twenty

Gratitude Isn't a Gimmick Because This Shit Can Always Get Worse.

"When it rains, look for rainbows; when it's dark, look for stars."

—Oscar Wilde

I can hear some of you already: What the fuck do I have to be grateful for? I've got cancer.

I hear you. Life dealt you the shittiest of hands, and finding things to be grateful for can seem an effort in futility. And some days your woe-is-me energy will be HIGH.

But stewing about the bad luck won't help you.

Gratitude is your brain's superpower.

Robert Emmons, author of *Gratitude Works*, wrote, "In fact, it is precisely under crisis conditions when we have the most to gain by a grateful perspective on life. In the face of demoralization, gratitude has the power to energize. In the face of brokenness, gratitude has the power to heal. In the face of despair, gratitude has the power to bring hope. In other words, gratitude can help us cope with hard times."[54]

How does this work?

Emmons argues that there's scientific evidence that grateful people are more resilient to stress, minor or severe, and cope in better ways during difficult times. Gratitude, he said, is a key

---

[54] Robert Emmons, "How Gratitude Can Help You Through Hard Times," *Greater Good Magazine*, May 13, 2013.

building block to our psychological immune systems and helps us bounce back faster.

It can also help while we're in the trenches fighting cancer.

How can I be grateful?

The simplest way I found to be grateful during my cancer treatment was reminding myself that, no matter how dark and bleak things were, they could always be worse. I could be waiting for diagnostic results in the middle of a war zone. Rather than *me* battling cancer, it could be someone dear to me instead. I *had* access to clean water, hospitals, doctors, and the like. Many people around the world do not. And no matter how terrible the battle seemed that particular day, I was still *alive*, and that was the most important victory of all.

I had a wonderful network of supportive family and friends, and many people do not. I was immensely grateful for all the people who showed up in my life during my time of need, and was continually touched by the thoughtfulness and deep care so many showed me at that time.

And the research studies were right. The more I focused on the things I was deeply grateful for, the more I told the universe *thank you*—for the nurse who held my hand during the biopsy, for PJ who came to every doctor's appointment with me, for the sister-in-law who sent me a funny care package filled with an irreverent pair of socks and a journal with the cover "I hear your titties are being shitty", and for the friend who sent me weekly little pick-me-up gifts during chemo to show I was in her thoughts—the more I felt *better*.

I feel it's just this: that despair feeds on feeling alone and unloved. The more I focused on the reality that I was *not* alone and I *was* loved, the harder it was for despair to take hold. The harder it was to feel despondent and depressed because I'd created a long and growing list of the things I was grateful for, the *good* things in my life.

If you're looking for good news, you'll find it.

This is a glass-half-empty kind of argument. If you're looking for terrible news, for confirmation that you're worthless, you don't fit in, and the world hates you, you'll find it. We never run out of bad stuff to pile into our brains (remember that negative playlist from Chapter Eighteen?).

Sometimes, and especially during cancer treatment, finding the silver lining can feel like mining precious minerals on an asteroid in space. Almost impossible.

But if you get in the habit of looking for the good, instead of the bad, you'll find the good news, too. And I believe the universe—God, or whomever you believe in—wants the best for you.

I don't believe the old adage, "God only gives you what you can handle." I think that's a load of bullshit. But I DO believe that in your darkest moments, the universe will sometimes give you a little boost, perhaps when you need it the most, and show you that there are better times ahead if you just hang on.

After my double mastectomy, before my chemotherapy, I was in a dark place. I didn't want chemotherapy. I was terrified of feeling nauseous all the time, worried about going bald, and just generally uneasy about voluntarily poisoning myself. The week before I was set to begin treatment, my husband took me to see the band Dogstar. For those who don't know, this is mega superstar Keanu Reeves' band (he plays bass), and I've been a HUGE Keanu Reeves fan for decades. I love his movies, but even more than that, I love his kindness and charity to others. My fandom is so well known in my family that when I was diagnosed with cancer, instead of sending flowers, my mom sent me a life-sized cardboard cutout of Keanu Reeves because she knew that would buoy my spirits more than daisies ever would.

As the opening notes of the first song began and the stage lights went up, Keanu began playing his bass, and the audience erupted in screams of joy and excitement. I don't even remember the songs they played, but I do remember feeling pure joy. I was standing in the same room as my idol! And it felt like, for just a brief moment, the universe shone a light on me. That the universe was saying, *We know you're going through it. Here's something good. Something purely wonderful. Just for you. Keep going. Life is worth living, and there will be more joyful moments like this on the other side of chemo.*

I really felt that was the message as I stood in the crowd, and I was completely and utterly overcome by gratitude. For that moment, for that blissful moment of joy, it was all the more amazing BECAUSE I was in the middle of the battle of my life. Tears of joy burned my eyes, and I kept sending up a silent prayer of thanks. I was so, so grateful because I needed this little lift so much. This was a special magical moment just when I needed it most.

"I've heard the expression about cloud nine, but I've never seen it before you. I've never seen anyone float like you did that night," my husband said later.

And I've thought about it some since then. I've also thought about all the amazing coincidences that lined up to allow me to be in that auditorium when I was.

I've been a Keanu Reeves fan for decades. I tried to see his band Dogstar when they last toured (with no luck getting tickets). His band broke up during the COVID pandemic, and then, right before my cancer diagnosis, they got back together, released a new album, and went on tour during the very year I had breast cancer. Despite a year of nonstop procedures and tests, the concert date just happened to be perfectly situated in between my surgery and my first chemo treatment—in the very small window when I'd recovered enough from surgery to go out and not yet sick from chemo treatments to want to stay in.

Think of the stars that had to align right at that moment so that I could see Keanu, right at the moment I needed a boost.

Now I know many of you feel like this was just happenstance and coincidence, and that's fine. But I chose to believe the universe was looking out for me—and I got a little boost when I desperately needed it—that would help me make it through chemo.

You might not be seeing Keanu Reeves, but if you look around you, you might see the universe trying to do the same thing for you. You might see that you ARE loved and you are not alone; good things are coming your way, even in the middle of all this bad. And even more—you DESERVE these good things and they'll make you feel grateful.

Everything seems like it's trash. How do I start being grateful?

Write three things you're grateful for every day in a journal. They don't have to be big things, they can be small. Some of mine were *very* small. (I'm grateful for hot water in my shower. Hell, I'm grateful for showers in general. I'm grateful for apricot jam. I'm grateful for my favorite song.)

Sometimes, when everything seems overwhelmingly terrible, focusing on very small things can help you get through.

Plenty of research shows that we can rewire our brains to be more grateful by short journal entries focused on gratitude.[55] You may have tried this when you were well and found it hard to do.

Things may feel hopeless, and you may wonder: how can I feel grateful when I lack all hope?

One thing researchers found that worked for some was to ask them to think about a time they were hopeful about something, and it DID work out.

Was it that time you were hopeful you'd get the promotion and you did?

That time you were hopeful you could go on that vacation and you did?

Maybe you had a crush on someone. . . and it turned out they had a crush on you right back.

Maybe, a long time ago, you were hopeful you could get into a particular college, and you did.

It's easy in bad times to go back through your life and think: Everything is awful, and everything has always been awful. Your luck is shit, and you've got a long list of all the times you lost hope or were disappointed or blindsided with bad news.

But good things happened as well. You wished for good things, and they happened. Researchers found that when people focused on a time in their lives when they were hopeful AND their hopes were realized, they felt better and more hopeful *in the present*.[56]

---

[55] Yu Komase, Kazuhiro Watanabe, Daisuke Hori, Kyosuke Nozawa, Yui Hidaka, Mako Iida, Kotaro Imamura, Norito Kawakami, "Effects of gratitude intervention on mental health and well-being among workers: A systematic review," Journal of Occupational Health, November 2021.

[56] Amy Morin, "How to Develop Hope When You Feel Hopeless," *Psychology Today*, June 25, 2023.

Do you think it's harder to find good news? Harder to find those good memories now in this terrible present? I think the opposite is true.

When you've got a whole lot of bad news, it's easier to celebrate the good.

It'll be *easier*, not *harder* to feel grateful right now. This sounds counterintuitive. How can this be? I've got cancer, I'm a human pin cushion, and none of my diagnostic tests are coming back the way I want!

When life deals you a shit sandwich, then you are MUCH more grateful when it gives you actually decent fries as a side. Thank goodness for those fries. You wouldn't be able to live without them! The same is true for good news of any kind that comes your way right now. Your kid got into the college they want? You're DOUBLY happy and relieved. Your favorite celebrity followed you back on socials? Let's shout that from the rooftops. You woke up after your tenth round of chemo actually feeling semi-human? It's time to fucking celebrate.

And let's not forget that most of the treatments many of you will have will be temporary. When radiation ends, you can throw yourself a huge-ass party in your brain. THAT is good news. When any horrible stage of this fight ends, that is good news and worthy of gratitude.

In this trying time, gratitude can find you in ways it can't when things in your life are going well. When you're facing cancer, every time you escape death, it's easy to feel grateful. When you finally get good news—from a scan or test—you will feel the weight of the dread of bad news you'd been carrying lift, and your heart will automatically be filled with gratitude.

Oh, thank God.

You WILL find yourself saying these words at one point or another because good news WILL eventually come your way.

The FUCKING DRAINS will come out—*Thank God.* The radiation will end—*Thank God.* The limbo of not knowing what the plan of treatment will be replaced with a plan of action. *Thank God.*

You'll be sending up prayers of thanks without even thinking about it.

So at this time, cultivate that gratitude. Help it grow. Gratitude makes you stronger because it reminds you you're loved and not alone. That the universe and the people who care about you are looking after you.

And you'll need that love and care more than ever.

Pep talk #20:
Hey, Badass. Today is the day you'll find something to be thankful for, thank goodness. When the night is darkest, that's when you see the most stars. All you have to do is find the first one. Once you find the first bright dot in the sky, you'll suddenly see more. And more. And more.

The gratitude you feel in your heart will grow, and it will be an engine, a power source for you. You will be able to cut down doubt and dread at the knees with gratitude. Feeling genuinely grateful will help raise you up. Gratitude is your secret weapon.

Chapter Twenty-One
Death—The Original Big D Energy

"Death is not the opposite of life, but a part of it."

—Haruki Murakami

Hi, warrior. You're fighting to live, so why do you want a chapter about Death?

Because we're all running from it, trying to deny it's ever really coming for us, but you don't have the privilege to do that anymore. Now you have to face Death, and Death is the original Big D energy.

When I was diagnosed, I suddenly saw death everywhere. At the infusion center. In the cancer treatment waiting room. In the bathroom mirror. In that fucking windowless room with the round table. In the warning hazard labels on the chemo bags.

And whether you're Stage 1 or Stage 4 (though especially if you're Stage 4), Death has become friendly with you, and you don't like it. He's standing in your lawn with a boom box overhead or stalking you on social media. He's come to your house, pretending to be a Christmas caroler, when he really just wants to show you a bunch of cue cards, putting you in the awkward position of knowing he's in love with you, the wife of his best friend, a la *Love Actually*.

I didn't say Death was classy.

But he is single-minded, and eventually, he comes for us all. Eventually, it won't be a distant crush or a minor stalking. He'll come for us. All of us. Some of us sooner rather than later, and there's really nothing any of us can do about it. We can try to put him off. We can delay him. We can postpone. But eventually, he's coming.

We all know death is inevitable, but few of us live our lives with this truth.

Before your cancer diagnosis, I'm guessing you didn't spend a lot of time thinking about death. You made plans, organized vacations, and you let yourself get drowned in the petty bullshit we often distract ourselves with every day of our lives (workplace scuffles, fretting about how we look, tolerating inconsiderate friends).

You did this because you were 30 or 40 or 50 or 60 or however old you were and thought you had the luxury of time. And now, with cancer, you see starkly that time is a precious resource that you might have frittered away. What would you give right now to have *more time*, to get back all the time you wasted doing all the things that weren't that important after all. Cancer is the biggest wake-up call. Cancer puts everything into stark focus: You are mortal. You will die. And death will almost always come sooner than we want.

In America, we go to great lengths to avoid talking about death.

"We don't die well in America," journalist Bill Moyers said in 2000. He did a whole series on PBS called "Living with Dying." In it, Moyers said, "Like you, I don't want to think about death—especially my own. But I have realized that death is pushing through the door we try to keep so firmly shut. Parents age before our eyes. AIDS and cancer take friends and loved ones. And baby boomers. . . face their own mortality even as they must care for their elderly parents. So like it or not, we cannot push death back through the door."

Some suggest this is because dying goes against the American ideals of striving, succeeding, clinging to our youth.

We Use Distractions Not to Think About Death

But we don't want to think about death, so we ignore it. We deny it.

In America, eighty percent of people make a birth plan, but only twenty-two percent of people make a death plan.[57]

We are Olympic athletes at avoiding thinking about death.

We fear death so much that we spend a lot of time doing things that we think stave off the Grim Reaper. Ask a man who dates a woman half his age whether he's afraid of death or not (spoiler—he's the MOST afraid). Ask an older woman who sinks her entire paycheck into youth creams and plastic surgery whether she's afraid (she's also terrified). We go to some pretty extremes NOT to age, not to even let the concept of our own decline into our minds, that we spend most of our waking hours in denial.

If we just diet hard enough, work out long enough, get enough Botox, date younger and younger, then we won't age, we won't die, and we'll live forever, so we never have to make any tough decisions about how we spend this blink of time we get on earth.

We love to distract ourselves from death. We love to tell ourselves it won't happen to *us*, and certainly not before we're ninety.

We Fear Death So Much That We Create Stories to Tell Ourselves It Doesn't Matter

You can be spiritual, and I'm not going to get into anyone's beliefs right here—I respect them all. But I will say that we, as a species, fear death so much that almost all our religions explain Death away. They tell us where we'll go after we leave this earth, and that makes us feel okay with dying because we

---

[57] Lawrence R. Samuel Ph.D., "The Psychology of Death," *Psychology Today*, March 8, 2019.

have a story (I'm not judging anyone's beliefs) to tell ourselves about what happens when we get there. You can fervently believe your story is the correct story, and I certainly hope it is! We don't know for sure, and all of us simply have to act based on faith.

And if you are deeply religious—regardless of your religion—lean on that faith. It's wonderful and it's healing. That said, I don't know of any religion that tells you to skip over the living of this life, to just lie dormant waiting for Death to take you to the Afterlife. I don't know of any religion that tells you: "Do petty bullshit all day because you're just waiting out the clock."

Because this life, the right now, is the only thing we really have control over. We don't know for certain what happens to us when we die. Or what form we take in the afterlife. All we know is that right now, we're alive.

Fear of death can make us do dumb things.
A 2016 study found that the more we fear death, the more violent we can get.[58] The more we fear death, the studies say, the more likely we are to endorse revenge on our enemies or political violence. We lash out at others because we're afraid of dying, but we don't want to admit it.

Remember when we talked about fear shutting off our logical brain? Well, there's no greater fear than the fear of dying, and that short-circuits every logical thought.

Think of the bully on the playground. The bully is almost always extra violent because they're afraid. That's why they

---

[58] Hirschberger, Gilad, Pyszczynski, Tom, Ein-Dor, Tsachi, Shani Sherman, Tal, Kadah, Eihab, Kesebir, Pelin, Park, Young Chin, "Fear of death amplifies retributive justice motivations and encourages political violence," *Peace and Conflict: Journal of Peace Psychology*, February 2016.

pick the weakest kid to pick on, because they definitely don't want to pick on anyone who could actually cause them harm. They thrive when the odds are in their favor. That's why, when you confront a bully head-on, they usually leave you alone.

Alok, a comedian, believes a lot of hateful rhetoric in society right now comes down to our fear of dying. "Transphobia is merely a distraction from our shared humanity," Alok said. "We should be talking about the fact that we're all going to fucking die."

On an appearance on *The Daily Show*, the comedian elaborated on this sentiment.

"I'm going to die and you're going to die, and we've created a society that pretends that that's not the case, which is just ridiculous," Alok said. "So people keep on thinking that if they imbibe the blood of their like eighteen-year-old son, they can stave off death, or like find the next cryptocurrency or something, but, girl, you're gonna die. You know what I'm saying? So actually, the real biological truth in our society is our mortality."

Grief makes us afraid to think about death.

I had a friend who lost their spouse to cancer. This friend's world was turned upside down from grief when they were left to be a single parent to small children. Grief felt so huge for this friend that they could no longer read or see any romantic comedies because sometimes there'd be death in these stories— death of a parent or death of a partner – and the very idea of thinking about death at all felt overwhelming. So they'd apologize to me—they'd written off an entire genre of movies and fiction for fear they might run into death.

I didn't blame this friend.

Grief is overwhelming. It does what it wants, and the more powerful the love, the more powerful the grief. Grief, after all, is just the loss of love. Grief shows up when it wants, and it does what it wants. And the only way to work through grief is to acknowledge it.

Part of what's so scary about grief is that we worry that death changes our relationship. That if our loved one dies, then that means it erases our love. But Death doesn't end a relationship.[59]

The relationship and the love continue—even when the person dies. If your parent or grandparent died, did you stop loving them because their physical bodies weren't here? No, of course not. Did you stop loving your amazing dog just because he crossed the rainbow bridge? No, you didn't. Do they—even though they're not physically here anymore—stop loving you? No. Of course, not.

I think of love as energy. The first law of thermodynamics is that energy in the universe can't be created, and it can't be destroyed. It simply is converted from one form to another. Love can't be destroyed, either.

So, those relationships continue. Physical death doesn't change our emotional relationship. Death doesn't have the power to take love away.

You love people who are not physically here anymore. And people will continue to love you when you aren't here anymore, too. All that you will truly leave when you're gone is the love in people's hearts that you planted there.

Make it a bumper crop.

Other countries and cultures don't run from death as hard as Americans do.

In other countries, like Austria, people don't run away from death. They in large part embrace it as a part of life.

---

[59] Lani Leary Ph.D., "Death Does Not End a Relationship," *Psychology Today*, July 12, 2012.

Last summer, our family went to Vienna. We traveled there because two of our children had a school trip that ended there, and we met them to extend the trip. In Vienna, death isn't avoided. It's celebrated. There's a deep and beautiful funeral culture there. People spend their lives planning elaborate tombstones, thinking about different aspects of their funerals, and even celebrating all aspects of burial in a funeral museum. Sigmond Freud didn't understand this preoccupation with death and called it, "death mania," but if you're ever in Vienna, do yourself a favor and visit the Central Cemetery.

Not only are some of Vienna's most famous former residents buried there (Beethoven and Brahms to name two), but the monuments and mausoleums there are gorgeous works of art. An army of groundskeepers work tirelessly day and night shining and cleaning the tombstones—which come in an amazing variety—classical, modern, dark, light, with sculptures and engravings and poems. Beethoven's grave looks brand new, as pristine as if he were buried yesterday. You cannot tell which graves are new or old, and everyone tells a unique story about the person's life. Musicians, artists, and businesspeople use the monuments and stones at their graves to tell a story of how they lived.

The cemetery is such a popular destination that a café sits at the entrance, so people can drink coffee and eat cake before or after their visit. The living and the dead coexist in a way there that they simply don't in most American cities.

In America, we think of cemeteries more often than not as a backdrop to horror movies, as creepy and dusty, and places that are neglected because we work strenuously to avoid them. Not in Vienna. Cemeteries are—as they should always be—a celebration of life, a place where death is as natural as breathing, and the whole point of living is to live so well you have a life worth remembering.

THERE'S NO GOOD BOOK FOR THIS

People pivot hard when it comes to death.

Remember when we told people that we had cancer and we got the pity and pivot? If we tell them the cancer is far advanced and we might die, let me tell you, they REALLY don't want to talk about it. They don't know what to say and they don't know what to feel. Let's be real—neither do we. There are a few TED talks out there discussing how we need to be brave listeners when people tell us something we don't want to hear.

Did you know there's a whole industry around dying?

Did you know there are death doulas? People who help guide you to the end?

There are resources out there and advocates: endwell project.org.

There are experts that can guide us through: inelda.org.

And it's also important to note that planning for death, and talking about death, doesn't bring the end any sooner. It just helps you meet the end on your own terms.

Dr. Kathy Kortes-Miller wrote a book for Canadians called *Talking About Death Won't Kill You: The Essential Guide to End-of-Life Conversations* where she walks you through a whole host of ways you can think about and plan for death.

"From the moment we are born, our cells are dying and they continue to do so throughout our life. So if dying is always a part of our living," Kortes-Miller said in a Ted Talk in 2016, "doesn't it only seem logical then that we spend some time thinking about it, planning for it, and talking about it? And just maybe that will help us to live life more fully."

What if instead of avoiding death, we face it?

A cancer diagnosis, no matter what the stage, forces you to face your own mortality in a way that most people don't have to. It's a slow-moving, near-death experience, with plenty of weeks and months to digest what's happening to you.

And I know Death is terrifying. But what if we decide that the only true way to be okay with dying is to live your life the way *you* think is important. If you're a nurturer, then that means to nurture those around you. If you're a doer, that means DO the things that matter to you. If you're an observer, that means to observe and chronicle the heck out of life. If you're a creator, then, go fucking CREATE! WHO are you? WHAT kind of mark do you want to leave on this world? HOW do you want to be remembered?

Blast Beyoncé's song, "I Was Here" and get TO it.

For those of us facing death, *really* facing it, and those of us who still have time left on the clock—no matter how much time that is—we can use it. We can use it to live life to its fullest. To give love to those around us. To make a positive mark on the world. To *nurture*, or *do*, or *observe*, or *chronicle*, or *create*.

We might have a few weeks, a few months, or decades left to live in our lives, but it's never too late to do what we're meant to do. It's never too late to create or nurture or be the person we want to be.

Here's a little secret—it's not too late to focus on the things in life that matter. Some people never get the opportunity—even for an hour or a day—to realize and truly focus on what's important. Facing Death is terrifying, but it's also freeing. If you face Death, if you accept it as inevitable, and if you put aside whatever Afterlife you think is waiting for you— just put that aside for a minute—then it gives you the ability to focus on the now. On what you can accomplish or do or feel this minute. This hour. Today.

If the chemo, the radiation, or the surgery buys you another month, or another year, or another three decades of life, what are YOU going to do with it? Are you going to plop yourself back into your existence where you were focused on petty, small bullshit? Are you going to tolerate people who abuse you, belittle you, or do not value you? Or are you going to get in tune with the reason you were put here to begin with? If the chemo isn't going to work, and you want to stop, how are you going to live out the remainder of your life on your own terms?

Everyone feels there's a different purpose to life, but I believe that mine is to love others, shine light where I can, ease suffering (I write stories to give people hope and joy), be kind to others, and to LIVE, baby, *live*. It means appreciating the talents of others—through live music, art, and stories. It means taking my responsibilities—to my kids, my family, my friends, my dog, and my community—seriously. It means showing UP, always, because why waste a single minute dodging and hiding? If everyone *showed up*, then the world would be such a better place. So I'm showing up. Where I can. When I can. Because I don't have forever, and I only get so many opportunities.

Death is Not Defeat.

While I want you to fight your heart out to end cancer, I also want you to know that death is not—nor has ever been—defeat. Death is simply inevitable.

My mom likes to say, "We all get the time we get. And none of us get out of here alive."

I'll fight like hell to be here, but when it's my time to go? It's my time to go. Death isn't defeat. Living a life devoid of purpose, or a destructive life, or a selfish, petty, sociopathic life? THAT'S true defeat.

No matter who you think judges us at the end, or whether we even get judged, live your life in the way you feel brings meaning. Don't sweat the small stuff. Try not to get dragged into petty battles. Use your time to be kind, to do good, and try to avoid being an asshole. The world has enough of those already.

I strongly believe that death is just a door. It takes us to the next place we're supposed to be. We are that energy in thermodynamics that can't be created or destroyed—we just convert to something else. That next dimension or place where we go can be whatever you believe it to be. Maybe it's heaven. Maybe we're reincarnated into a different life. Or maybe we're just absorbed back into the energy of the universe. It doesn't mean we failed somehow because everyone has to go through that door, and we don't usually get to choose exactly when that time is.

Because Our Lives End, They Have Meaning

If we were to live forever, then, let's be honest, the things we do would matter less. If we had eternity to do whatever we wanted, then what makes life special? There'd be no urgency to do anything. And who would really care—if we never died, then we'd have eternity to work out life's big questions, if we chose to at all.

Our lives have meaning because we have a finite amount of time to walk this earth, in this body, on this plane, and make our mark. It's because we only have a certain amount of time on the clock that we can actually do some pretty amazing things.

"The way to value life, the way to feel compassion for others, the way to love anything with greatest depth is to be aware that these experiences are destined to be lost," writes Irvin D. Yalom in his book *Staring at the Sun: Overcoming the Terror of Death.*

In this book, he delves into ways we can overcome the fear we all carry of our lives ending, and ways we can prepare ourselves for the inevitable. He's a huge proponent of connection because, after all, making connections with others can give purpose and meaning to our lives, and he also urges readers to live their lives so that they have the fewest regrets by the end.

Existentialist Julian Barnes suggests in his quite funny memoir, *Nothing to Be Frightened Of*, that a fear of death goes hand in hand with our fear that we simply didn't live our lives well enough. We had always *meant* to get to all that important stuff we'd planned to do, but we got caught up in silly stuff, and when Death comes knocking, we just want a little more time. The best way to short-circuit this concern is to start living your life right now with the fewest regrets. Stop talking yourself out of the things you believe will make your life meaningful and start doing them. Now. With what time you do have left.

Pep talk #21:
Hey, Mortal Human.

Death comes for us all. We want to ignore that fact. But it's true.

You know Death's been stalking you. Eventually, he'll get you.

But he doesn't decide how you live, and he certainly doesn't decide how you face death. You get to decide these amazing things: how you live what life you have left, and how you face what comes for all of us.

Live your life with purpose and clarity and joy with the time—however much you have. Nobody gets out alive, so make the most of the time.

Live your life so you have no regrets.

Chapter Twenty-Two

Hey Spouses and Partners—It's Rough in the Passenger Seat. I See You.

"Cancer affects all of us, whether you're a daughter, mother, sister, friend, coworker, doctor, or patient."

—Jennifer Aniston

"Courage starts with showing up and letting ourselves be seen."

—Brené Brown

Hi, caregivers—spouses, partners, all of those medical powers of attorney—I see you.

It's been *rough* out here for you, I know it has.

Rougher even than us.

Because we've been raving lunatics with mood swings more violent than Linda Blair in *The Exorcist*. We're dealing with the fight of our lives, and all you can do is sit on the sidelines, hoping, like an anxious parent at the Olympics, that we don't break our necks on the vault. We're the ones who have to do all the heavy lifting, all the suffering, all the work. Cheering from the sidelines is a thankless and almost impossible job.

I see you.

You're doing great. Really. Even when we bite your heads off. (Wanna know why? Because we have fucking cancer, and we can't bite *its* head off. We're scared to death, and you're our safe spot to be angry—so we apologize for that). On behalf of all of us, let me tell you, *I'm sorry for what I said when I had cancer.*

Thank you. For being there.

We know that you got a whole lot of new responsibilities during our cancer treatment. You may have gone from doing 10% of the housework to 100%. You may have gone from doing 60% of childcare to 90%. You may have gone from earning 50% of the household income to 100%.

This sucks.

We know.

And on top of all that, you're supposed to be the Number One Cheerleader. The "You got this!" person when nothing you say seems exactly right.

Oof.

It's rough. We know.

And the worst part of all is that you can't just FIX IT.

There are many spouses out there who JUST WANT TO FIX IT.

Leaky faucet? I'll fix it.

Flat tire? I'll fix it.

This is not one of those things you can fix.

You'll want to. But you can't.

This is what sucks about being a caregiver. You can't fix anything. What you can do is ask, "What can I do to help?"

That's it.

You can help. You can't fix.

And you know what? Helping can be even better than fixing. It can be amazing and fulfilling and awesome.

The Lymph Node Is Benign

"Oh, thank God." My husband's shoulders literally sag, as if he's put down a deadlift weight bar. "Thank God." He pulls me into the warmest hug ever (PJ is great at hugs. If there were a gold medal in hugs, he'd win it every Emotional Olympics).

"I didn't realize. . . I didn't realize how heavy a load I'd been carrying. My God." He exhales and then pumps a fist in the air and claps three times. "This is what I'm talking about. Finally. Good news."

I didn't realize until right then what a stiff upper lip PJ had been sporting. That while I'd been on the terrifying rollercoaster of cancer, screaming my head off, he'd been right next to me trying to be brave for me, squeezing my hand, and keeping his face neutral, when inside he was screaming his head off, too.

"Those messy bitches didn't get their Uber," I say. "They're still stuck at the first bar."

PJ grins at me, relief clear on his face. "Good. They're going to stay there, too!"

Cancer causes collateral emotional damage to the whole family.

Cancer isn't a solo sport, at all. It's a team sport. When one person—especially a parent—gets cancer, it affects the entire family.

Studies show that relatives of those going through cancer treatment are more likely to be stressed out and more prone to depression than in healthy families.[60] Cancer brings all kinds of stress and emotional whiplash. Not only can treatment be dire, but the patient or caregiver can lose a job or income, giving the family something else to worry about. Not every job comes with paid medical leave.

My teen kids told me *after* treatment how stressful it had been for them, when they were all trying to keep a brave face.

---

[60] "Psychosocial Impact of Cancer Patients on Their Family Members" by Sun Min Lim, Hyeon Chang Kim, Soohyeon Lee, Division of Medical Oncology, Department of Internal Medicine, Yonsei University College of Medicine, Seoul, Korea.

That cancer had touched nearly every part of their life: friends, school, work.

Spouses are closest to the patient, so they often get a front-row seat to the horrors of diagnosis and treatment, and yet few people ask how *they're* doing. Everyone asks about the cancer patient, as they should, but then few remember to check in with the main caregivers—even the caregivers themselves. They don't have the cancer, but the person they love most in the world does.

It's just as terrifying for caregivers as for patients.

We're not the only ones scared shitless. You are, too. You don't want to be left trying to figure out what the hell we're having for dinner! Or who's on duty when the lonely freshman in college calls. Or what do you even DO on the holidays? (How do you wrap presents AND do all the baking? For Fuck's sake)

No matter where you are in your partnership, I'm guessing you never thought you'd be the one to outlive your spouse or that you'd have to deal with this kind of curveball.

Your instinct, no doubt, will be to hide, to avoid the doctor's appointments, to tune out when all the horrible treatments are presented. You'll want to tune out because it's simple self-preservation at work. If you tune in, then you might have to face the fact that this shit is really happening, so if you don't pay attention, or you hide, or you avoid, then maybe you can simply skip the terrible part and tune back in when everything is hunky dory.

Don't give into this temptation.

We need you.

Even when we say we've got it and we don't need you, we do.

We're going to be shaken. We're going to cry. We're going to think that whatever horrible thing is happening—surgery, chemo, radiation—this is our New Forever. Your job is to remind us that it isn't. That this temporary. That you will get back to a Better Normal. That it won't be horrible forever because nothing is. That you're in it together, and whatever horrible thing is coming down the pike, that she's got you by her side, and you'll face it together.

This is the best and biggest gift you can give your spouse.

Your partner will also want to hide. Encourage them not to.

Your partner might also want to hide away from you, worried that if you see the Terrifying Phonebook or if you see her hideous (actually Kick Ass Bravery Medal) scars that you won't find them attractive again.

They're worried you won't see them the same way.

And you won't. You'll now see them as a badass mother-fucking warrior who faced down their fear and kicked cancer's ass. Tell her that. That's sexier than ANY nipple anywhere on earth. Because, you have had a front row seat to the TERRIFY-ING journey that is a cancer battle, and you've seen her step into the fight every time.

It's up to you to show them that you're not that shallow. You love them for them, not their boobs. They're more than that to you. They are your partner, your best friend, your lover, and the person who means more to you than any other person in the world. Show them that.

Now is the time to show your partner how much they mean to you. Respect their wishes, always, but also show up in ways that make them comfortable confiding in you and sharing their insecurities.

Show your own vulnerability and maybe they will show you theirs.

Some people think being a supportive spouse means that you've got to be STRONG all the damn time. That you've got to not show that any of this is getting to you, or that you're scared, or that you don't know what to do. That you've got to hide your bad feelings, your fear, your anxiety, your doubt.

Show it ALL.

Be vulnerable.

What good are the fucking emotional walls doing? They're only keeping us out.

We don't really need a superhero who doesn't feel pain and who's impervious to bullets. We need the person we married to see us, be in it with us, and show us that it's okay to be scared or mad or frustrated because they are feeling the exact same things.

It's also okay to tell us that you don't know what to do.

NONE of us know what the fuck to do!

And I'll be honest—it's better to admit you don't know than to bluster and bluff, feeding us bullshit. Don't, whatever you do, mansplain cancer treatment.

EVERY fucking one of us had to stop and ask for directions because Google Maps does not provide an alternative route for this shit.

You have strong opinions, but the ultimate decision is not yours.

You may have a very strong opinion about a course of treatment or reconstruction, but I'm sorry to inform you, the choice is really ours. And that's how you're going to WANT it to be. This is life-changing, body-shifting stuff, and WE have to be bought into the decision and the treatment. It needs to be ours.

Be a sounding board, of course. Be supportive. But if you think this is your chance to get those double DDs you've been eyeing, then you do NOT have your head in the game.

Keep showing up.

We might tell you that you don't need to come to the doctor with us. We might say we don't need you to cook tonight. We might tell you all kinds of things.

Keep showing up. You're going to feel like your task list is impossible. That you can't do it all. And do you know what? You probably can't. Do the best you can. That's all.

You might also need to delegate. Do YOU really need to unload the dishwasher, or can the kids do it? Do you REALLY need to take on that extra project at work?

Remember, you've got the Cancer Card by proxy, and you can use it, too. "My spouse has cancer" is a fantastic excuse for getting out of that sales conference in Toledo.

Cancer can make your relationship stronger, or it can break you apart.

Like any scuffle with adversity, now is the time to figure out whether you—as a couple—plan to battle it back-to-back or battle each other.

This is a choice you two have to make. And it's a choice that's made a million little times along the way. Do you cancel your golf trip with buddies to go to that biopsy appointment? Do you clear your calendar the week of surgery? Do you step into the fray—even if you know your partner will criticize the way you fold the damn towels—because it's the right thing to do, dammit?!

Is it you and your loved one against cancer? Or does cancer get to wiggle its way between you and break you apart?

Both happen, trust me.

Burnout is real.

You'll hit a wall sometime. Lean on family and friends who offer to help. Don't think you can go it alone. You WILL feel overwhelmed at times, and that's okay. You're only human.

Delegate. Accept people's offer for help.

You—and your spouse—will need it!

You can be depressed and anxious, too.

We, the cancer patients, don't have a monopoly on anxiety and depression.

Spouses and partners of cancer patients get depressed and anxious, too. This is just a fact. A Denmark study found suicide rates higher for spouses of cancer patients than spouses of healthy people.[61]

Counselors love to talk about the oxygen masks on the airplane. Remember them? The flight attendants always warn us to put our masks on first before we help others. Why? Because if we don't, we can pass out trying to help someone else, and then we become a problem instead of a Helper.

So—in these difficult times—don't forget to put your own mask on first. Take care of yourself. Talk to a counselor. Do self-care. Blow off steam. Make sure you don't become depressed and despondent. It's easy to do.

Don't forget to take care of you.

We come first, and so do our appointments and our treatments and everything. But don't forget to take care of you—sleep, eat right, exercise. Blow up aliens in that video game you love so much. Watch your favorite sports team. Grab a beer or coffee with friends. Blow off steam.

---

[61] Jennifer Benjamin, "Treating Cancer: Spouses Need Support, Too," Northwell Health.

You're dealing with stress, too, so why not hit that treadmill or those weights?

We need you in your BEST possible condition. We need to lean on you, and we need you steady, that means you've got to take care of YOU. Self-care isn't just for us right now. It's for you, too.

Because if you're not right, if you're not ready, how can we lean on you?

And also—it's okay to ask for help. You need it, too.

You may start to feel resentful. This is normal and okay.

Spouses can start to feel resentful for a whole host of reasons. Taking care of your partner is A LOT. You're asked to step up and DO A LOT. You also aren't necessarily rewarded with gratitude. You might be rewarded with a bad mood and sarcasm. The weight of your sacrifice (missed work, picking up the kids, getting the prescriptions) might go without the proper thanks.

Your partner is in their own world right now, and you feel on the outside. That nothing you do is getting the praise it deserves. This sucks. It does.

Also, your partner is getting all the emotional support and praise (she deserves it, of course) but you wouldn't mind a crumb or two of support now and again.

And then after all your hard work, your spouse may be feeling terrible, nauseous from chemo, and the last thing on earth they want is sex. Are you even a couple anymore? You try to tell yourself that this is temporary (it is) and everything will come back (it will), but part of you fantasizes about not having to be the Stand-Up Spouse anymore. You know you vowed in sickness and in health, but you just didn't think sickness would suck this bad.

It's okay.

PJ would sometimes joke that the worst decision I ever made was to get cancer. This was a joke. Clearly. No one *chooses* cancer. It was also his way of blowing off steam a little bit. His way of saying, "Hey, this route sucks! What address *did* you put into Waze again?"

It was also his way getting to a fundamental truth: He knew it wasn't my fault, but this path sucked anyway and he hated it. Just as much as I did.

What can you do?

There are things you can do to help you get through. First, know that caring for yourself is just as important as caring for your spouse. Then, try to:

- **Communicate.** I know you're rolling your eyes because everyone always shouts about communication, but talk honestly about your feelings. Yes, the two of you are going through the battle of your lives, but don't keep resentments bottled up forever where they'll fester. And for the love of God, please use "I" statements and not derogatory "you do this" statements. *I know you may not intend this, but I feel underappreciated* is a whole lot better than *You make me feel terrible all the time.*

- **Reach out to your own support group or counselors.** Some spouses are terrible at having their own support group, but, man, you will need yours. The group can be friends and relatives. I'd seriously consider a counselor. You're going to need to sort through all kinds of things yourself, and to be the best supportive partner you can be, you're going to need to be the best self YOU can be in order to be the best partner you can be. This means talking to others. My husband made friends in so many waiting rooms. He even texts a husband he talked to when I was getting my double-mastectomy. This shit is hard, and spouses need connections and support, too. You'll have your own fear and anger to work through, and sometimes the best way to do that is with other caregivers going through the same things you are.

- **Plan something awesome for post-treatment.** Maybe this is a road trip you two have always wanted to go on. Or a concert. Or a restaurant. Or maybe you two want to learn how to ballroom dance. Or take over your parents' old cabin at the lake. Make a plan about post-treatment, something you both can look forward to and dream about during the roughest stages of treatment. Having a plan for the future that you BOTH are excited about, and then that will help you focus on something past cancer treatment.

Keep in mind, the passenger seat may be bumpy, but it's also a place of honor.

PJ and I recently went to dinner with a mother whose twenty-something daughter developed a rare but aggressive form of bone cancer in her leg, which required the amputation of her foot, as well as chemotherapy and other treatments. Her mom stepped in to help take care of her during this time and the treatment was ROUGH. It was a grueling time, a difficult time, watching her baby girl lose her foot, her hair, and then become so weak she could barely smile, so nauseous she couldn't keep food down.

But when we talked with her and I mentioned this very book I was writing and how I wanted to include a chapter for caregivers because of how difficult and lonely that journey can be, she said, "I don't know how you feel, PJ, but it was an honor for me to care for her. I was honored to do it."

PJ emphatically agreed.

She went on to say that every time she picked up meds or carted her to chemotherapy treatments or doctor's appointments, she was grateful to be there, to be the one holding her hand. She loved her daughter so much, she wouldn't want anyone else there taking care of her, even if that meant having barf bags at the ready. She was glad to do it, honored to have the chance to do it.

When you're a caregiver, it's easy to get run down, to focus on the negatives, to start thinking you're not being appreciated enough. That's just human. But it IS an honor to care for someone you love. That's why marriage vows don't say, "In health and just all the fun or easy times." You didn't pledge love and loyalty to a partner because you knew life was easy. You did it *because* you know life is hard. Because we all need our person in times of trouble.

And cancer is big trouble.

We chose you. We want you there. Of all the people in our life, all the people we could've tapped to come to every appointment, to see us at our most vulnerable, we picked you.

We want you there.

We're honored to have you there by our side.

Pep talk #21:

Hey, warrior spouses and partners, thank you.

Thank you for being there for us. Thank you for picking up our slack.

Thank you for loving us, and for letting us know that we're beautiful in your eyes, no matter what. Thank you for standing with us in the storm, even when we're making the storm.

Remember that you're going through something here, too. You're suffering cancer's collateral damage.

It's not selfish to take care of you, so you can take care of us.

Be there for yourself so you can be there for us.

You've got this. We picked you for a reason, and we're so glad you're here with us.

Chapter Twenty-Three
Life After Cancer—
Why Don't I Feel Happier?

"Cancer is only going to be a chapter in your life, not the whole story."

—Joe Wasser

I know some of you will live with cancer your whole life. You will have treatments at the infusion center forever. I salute you, warriors. For you, the battle never ends.

For those of you who will beat down cancer until it's undetectable in your bodies, this is a special chapter for you.

Normal Life Feels Weird

You've had the battle of your life, and now you've come home. Everyone is normal, and everything seems great, except you've got PTSD and nothing seems right. Your friends and family will want to ring bells with you, throw confetti, toast you. And you'll celebrate.

But maybe. . . just maybe. . . this time feels. . . off.

Some people find the year after battling cancer to cause the most mental strain. At my last regular oncologist's appointment, before she let me go for six (whole!) months, she warned me that, post-cancer, many people face serious depression. Some women have a very hard time going back to their lives. Some women have problems adjusting.

You know why?

Because you spent the last year, fifteen, or twenty months in the fight of your FUCKING life. You were on the battlefield every fucking day, facing down DEATH, PAIN, and DISFIGUREMENT. You carry the scars of your wounds that you still probably haven't made full peace with, and everybody just wants to ring a bell, pat you on the back, and send you on your way, forgetting it ever happened.

Except you won't forget.

You carry the scars.

Maybe you have numbness. Maybe you have pain. Maybe you can't ever reach that damn high shelf again. Maybe you lost your nipples or all feeling in your chest. Maybe you burst into tears randomly all the time. Or maybe... like me... you see a white coat and your blood pressure goes straight through the roof.

It's a mind fuck. Have no doubt.

You're walking off a different kind of battlefield. You've been to a different kind of war. You've experienced something traumatic and horrible, and now you're told it's time to return to normal life. They're asking you to put down your weapons. And... what now?

It's okay NOT to be over cancer, even if it's not detectable in your body.

At this stage of my treatment, at the end, when there was no detectable cancer in my body and my immunotherapy was simply an insurance policy—though a painful one (you try having a nurse poke you five times looking for a vein for the IV)—I was supposed to be happy and relieved.

I played Taylor Swift's "Out of the Woods" because that's how I felt. *AM I out of the woods? When IS the other shoe going to drop?* Can I start to celebrate? Why does celebrating feel so wrong?

I'd faced so many twists and turns in this battle to take back my life, so many surprising setbacks (like, surprise, you SHOULD get chemo after all!), that part of me simply didn't believe the battle was over.

Cancer took up my full attention for fifteen months, and now. . . I didn't have to worry about it every second of every day? The messy bitch really *was* gone? I couldn't wrap my head around it.

Allow yourself time to adjust.

You're returning home from war. There WILL be an adjustment period, and that's okay.

If you haven't paid someone to listen to you, I suggest doing that now.

Fighting cancer is a kind of trauma all its own, and if you haven't processed it *while* it was happening, your brain will force you to process it all now.

Talk to a therapist.

Meditate.

Talk to your friends (the ones who aren't sick about hearing about it).

Join a survivors group—in person or online. Connect with people who've been through what you've been through.

Remember that it's okay to be frustrated with friends or colleagues who seem to be floating through life with zero understanding of how lucky they are NOT to have been battling cancer the last year.

But why am I not happier?

You spent all these months praying for this moment—to be officially cancer-free. What you wouldn't have given a year ago, to be set free into the world and told you're now, really, seriously, in remission. Cancer-free. Healthy. Ready to get back to your old life.

So. . . why don't you feel. . . happier?

Sure, I felt relieved. So relieved. But I was surprised that the news didn't make me. . . happy. Like the kind of fundamentally fulfilled. Like, what I imagined winning the lottery would feel like: Finally! I don't have to worry about anything ever again!

Except life doesn't work like that, exactly.

There's no goal accomplished that's a magic bullet that solves all your problems. There's still dinner to make. Grown children to worry about. College that your oldest must apply for. There are bills to pay (more than you had before), and if you're like me, you might've lost your job during your treatment.

Fun!

But still. Cancer-free. You did it! You're supposed to be happy.

But maybe you're not.

It sounds completely ungrateful, doesn't it? There are women who will go every week or every month to that damn cancer center for treatment for the rest of their lives. They won't ever be in remission. I should be grateful and celebrate, but remission didn't make me gleeful. My life was the same: work, run the kids around, try to finish that new manuscript, fret about money (especially with the added medical expenses), do a seemingly endless pile of dishes, try to get a new publishing contract, worry about that some more. Rinse. Repeat. The news of being cancer-free didn't transform my life. My life was. . . my life.

Sometimes reaching a goal can feel disappointing.

Sometimes, the journey is more satisfying than actually achieving the goal.

We spend a lot of our time fantasizing about reaching a particular goal and feeling like if we only get *there*, then our problems are solved.

Psychologists call this the Arrival Fallacy. The happiness guru Tal Ben-Shahr, who wrote *Happier*, coined the phrase. He told *The New York Times* that the Arrival Fallacy is the "illusion that once we make it, once we attain our goal or reach our destination, we will reach lasting happiness."

So, the Arrival Fallacy tells us that if we just work hard and reach our goal, then we'll finally, and at long last, be happy and content. It's a form of cognitive bias that tells us some future event, the reaching of some goal, will produce consistent and positive feelings in our life.[62]

And let's face it, beating cancer is one helluva goal. The noblest of goals.

You've been working your ass off to achieve this moment. If you can only get back to your old life, the one without the horrible, debilitating stress of cancer, then you'll be happy. THEN you will finally be grateful for all the things in your old life before cancer came. THEN you'll finally DO THE THING you always wanted to do, then you'll finally be. . . content and happy forever.

And the doctor gives you the all-clear.

And then everything is pretty much the same.

The clouds don't part and rainbows don't shoot out of your ass (if they do, then I definitely want to know what the hell kind of chemo you were on. Also, what fun you will be at parties)!

In his book *Happier*, Ben-Shahr says that, by focusing on a future goal, this triggers reward centers in the brain and helps us feel soothed. Meaning, the more we plan for something to happen and focus on a goal, the more our brain releases good

---

[62] "Arrival Fallacy: Why Success Isn't As Fun As You Expected?" *The Happiness Blog*, November 3, 2024.

chemicals, making us feel soothed and rewarded. The irony is, the more you focus on a goal, the more your brain rewards you with good chemicals along the way and your body adjusts to the good feeling of the goal. So when you actually achieve it, the good chemicals don't rush to you because you've been doling them out in small amounts this whole time.

You've been anticipating success this whole time. That means when it comes, you are oddly disappointed by it.

I suffered the Arrival Fallacy when I published my thirty-seventy book, *The Second You're Single* under my given name, Cara Tanamachi. Before that book, I'd been in series books with Harlequin. These are the pulpy paperback romance novels that are amazing, but also aren't single title trade paperbacks. There's a hierarchy in publishing. It goes: mass market paperback (smaller, less expensive), trade paperback (larger, more expensive), hardback (the most expensive).

I started my career in trade paperback, with a bestseller that became a Lifetime Original Movie *I Do (But I Don't)*. I wrote several more books for Simon and Schuster, only to get cut, and find myself wandering around for another contract. Novelists rarely have job security, unless you're one of the rare top-selling ones: Emily Henry, Nora Roberts, Kennedy Ryan, Stephen King. They're whole economies unto themselves.

So, I spent years publishing mass-market category romance, remanded to the back shelves of the bookstores (if I was in a bookstore at all, and not just online). I spent all my time thinking: if only I could get back to my former glory of trade paperback. If only I could. . .

And then I did.

I landed a two-book trade paperback deal.

And book one of that deal was published.

And I was happy. For a little while. But then, the happiness *didn't* last.

And then I started to realize that this one shiny goal I thought would make me complete didn't actually solve all my problems. I still butted heads with my then middle-school-aged daughter. I still didn't have the retirement savings I wanted. I still fretted about whether I could take time off, and I never lost those stubborn ten pounds I'd been trying to lose forever, and. . . the list went on and on.

And the short-lived happiness from the book being published faded because life started up again. It was just as it had been before, and then I just felt. . . sad. Disappointed. Empty. I'd been pedaling so hard to reach the finish line, and now that I was there. . . well, I still had most of my problems (minus the one about being published in trade paperback) and none of the sustainable bliss I could've sworn would've come from the accomplishment. And instead of feeling ecstatic. . . I started to feel disappointed. This was. . . it? This was. . . all? I'd put so much of myself to achieving this goal, SO many fucking hours, so much stress, so much effort. . . and now I had a nice book. On the shelf of a bookstore.

And, yes, it was a major accomplishment, and I was proud of it, but I realized I'd put so many expectations on making this ONE goal that I'd unconsciously began to believe that, if only *this* happened, then everything would fall into place in my life. That every single worry I ever had about my career would immediately evaporate, and I'd be left with a long-lasting, fulfilling peace that I'd always been seeking.

Yet, that didn't happen.

I published the book.

Life went on. And it wasn't the bubby, perfectly happy, amazing life I'd imagined after *just getting this one thing accomplished*. It was. . . well, life. Messy. Stressful. Busy. Wonderful, joyful, and amazing, but also terrible and disappointing and frustrating. It was. . . life. Sometimes, I overslept my alarm. Sometimes, I forgot things I should remember. Sometimes, people wrote bad reviews of my book, and sometimes they wrote good ones.

Publishing the single book was fantastic, amazing, and awesome, but it didn't solve all my problems. And now, because I achieved that goal, I didn't even have a bright, new, shiny goal at the ready to look forward to. To pine for. To dream about. I had to find a new goal. A new something to make me dream about how things could be better.

I felt the same about beating cancer.

You achieve your goal, your all-encompassing goal, and. . . well, now what? What do you do with the hours you don't have to spend at chemo? What do you do with the entire nights you aren't lying awake, staring at the ceiling and facing your own mortality (fun tip: you can still stare at the ceiling and worry about. . . anything. The grocery list you forgot to make. The utility bill you need to pay!). And what new dream/goal/achievement will help you feel better about your current life by just thinking about the what if. . .?

So—beating cancer doesn't solve all your problems. Of course, it doesn't. You know what it does? It takes a BIG FUCKING PROBLEM off your plate.

You still have life—in all of its messy glory—to live. Curing cancer wasn't going to bring you sustainable happiness. Living your life in a way that's true to you, who you are, who you want to be, and what you want to do with your remaining time on this planet, will bring you that contentment.

So.

What now?

It's time to find a new goal. A new dream. Something even better to focus your attention on. You've beat cancer, so now focus on what next.

The sooner you get that new goal in your mind, I promise you, the better you'll feel. Do you want to write a book? Change careers? Go back to school?

Now is the time to focus on a new goal.

We humans are strivers. We're always working towards the next big thing. So get to work on your next big dream. Your next accomplishment. Your next goal.

Do I need to make something meaningful out of this?

That's up to you. Many women do. They start charities. They raise money. They make networking groups. They follow research. They knit caps for chemo patients. They do all kinds of amazing things. They walk a bajillion miles for the Susan G. Komen Foundation. Or, like me, they write a book with a whole lot of F bombs.

You can do this, too.

Or, you don't have to.

That's the amazing part of all of this. Just like with how you decided to fight cancer. YOU get to decide how to live!

Do I need to start worrying about recurrence?

That's up to you. Your oncologist will give you the odds. It's up to you whether to let them take up real estate in your brain.

The specter of cancer will always hover across your life. This is a fact.

But if you've done everything in your power to fight it, then you've done what you can do. It's out of your hands. No sense wasting good worrying time on cancer, when you can worry about other things (Remember finances? Adult children without careers living in your basement? Passive-aggressive in-laws? Incompetent bosses? Societal injustice?). Those old familiar worries are still there, waiting for you. Why not give them a spin?

Plus, here's the bonkers thing: you can make actual, real sustainable changes in your life. You can eat better. You can walk more. You can drink less. You can give up smoking. You can do all these things. Because doing these things is easier than another round of cancer. Doing these things is a great way to channel that worry.

You stressed about recurrence? Good news. There are ways to tip the odds:[63]

- **Lace up those walking shoes and go for a walk.** Having a hard time getting motivated to do it? Tell yourself that walking is medicine. It's treatment. And it's a helluva lot easier treatment than getting chemo through an IV.
- **Eat right.** You don't have to be perfect, but getting rid of processed foods, fatty meats, and sugar can do wonders.
- **Drink less.** Nobody wants to hear this but it's true: three to four alcoholic drinks PER WEEK (not night) increase your chances of breast cancer, and the more you drink, the greater the risk.
- **Use less plastics, parabens, preservatives, and other toxic chemicals.** Once you've gotten cancer, everything seems like it's trying to kill you. There are plenty of apps that can help you track clean foods and beauty products. You can go down a very dark rabbit hole on this one. Do what makes sense to you. Remember, you can't control everything, and some things will get through. I think the important thing to remember here is balance. How can you *reduce* risk but also *live* your life and not obsess over every single chemical and microplastic?

---

[63] "How to Lower Your Risk of Breast Cancer Recurrence," University of Rochester Medical Center, October 18, 2022.

I still feel lost.

You might find the reintroduction to civilian life hard. The re-entry can be a bitch. There are things to do.

Join a support group. Sometimes, as you battle Arrival Fallacy, you might need to talk about this with others. Remember that it's okay to be disappointed that kicking cancer's ass isn't the silver bullet you thought it would be. It's okay to feel depressed or despondent. The goal itself was never going to bring you the happiness you seek. Only living your life, the way you want to live it, every day, will do that.

Talk to a counselor. The battle in your body might be over, but the battle in your mind might just be beginning.

Give yourself grace. Others will move on, but you've just come off the battlefield. OF COURSE, you will be jumpy and skittish. You will have PTSD.

Do things that bring you joy. The one lesson to learn from this shit show is that joy is fleeting, and bad news can drop into your life at any moment so *take advantage of every fucking healthy day.* Doing things you love isn't selfish. It's fucking necessary. Pack in those good memories, those good times, those things that bring you joy because you'll need those memories to keep you warm in the bad times. You've EARNED some fucking laughs. You've been through the dark times. Walk in the light and appreciate it all the more.

Pep talk #22:

Hey, Champion. You've climbed the mountain, but you can't enjoy the view. You thought you wouldn't need any more pep talks anymore, but you find you need them all just to keep going. That just means you're human. You put a lot into this moment of being cancer-free.

This fight is what you make of it. You get to decide what meaning—if any—to take from it. What I do know for sure is that you are a brave, badass motherfucker. Hold your head high.

Chapter Twenty-Four
Learn to Ignore Little Shit, and After Cancer? It's All Little Shit.

"Once I overcame breast cancer, I wasn't afraid of anything anymore."

—Melissa Etheridge

You've walked through a fucking blazing fire and come out the other side a motherfucking phoenix.

You deserve to celebrate. You deserve all the gold medals. You deserve all the standing ovations.

YOU did this. YOU made the hard calls. YOU took charge of your care. You fucking kicked cancer's ass.

With your new power of I AM IN CHARGE, *stay* in charge. Your life, what is left of it, is yours to fucking live. And guess what? You are a newly minted brave, tough, motherfucker. You CAN do scary things. Going after that promotion? Quitting your job? DO it. Is it scarier than radiation? Chemo? Getting your boobs cut off?

Hell, no, it's not.

The thing about staring death in the face is that you now know what others don't: time is precious. During all those treatments (especially chemo) I learned the hard way that plans are an illusion, that life is definitely what fucking happens when you're making plans. Even after cancer, plans are still an illusion.

We know more than anyone else that you never know when life is over—for any of us—and that hard truth always comes too soon.

At the end of your journey, when people tell you you're brave, you won't say, "Oh, it was nothing" or "I'm not brave." You will say, "I know I'm brave."

Because you fucking are.

You've walked through the fire and come out one smokin' hot bitch.

Because you know you will have faced down shit-your-pants inducing terror, and you will have let it wash over you until only you remain. You will have let fear shake that plane with the turbulence of a lifetime, but you kept your cool, and landed that plane safely on the ground.

When people say I'm brave, I don't shirk off the compliment. I *know* exactly what it took to get here. I *know* how shit-scared I was through the whole damn process. I know I was a bull in a china shop, and I KNOW how hard it was to keep going—through the nausea, the hair loss, the surgeries, the pain.

You want to say I'm brave? I know I am.

And you will know it, too.

You won't just think you can handle your shit, you *know* you can handle your shit.

There's something amazing in that, let me tell you. If there's any gift in cancer at all, it's that.

I've been confident in my life, sure, but I've also lived with an undercurrent of anxiety my whole life. I would get floating bouts of anxiety—like when I was just sitting in class or at my desk for work. I'd get butterflies for no reason at all.

I always worried—would I be able to handle x, y, or z? I always fretted about not living up to expectations (mine and other people's). I used to live in mortal fear of failure and humiliation.

I don't worry so much about that anymore.

I'm resilient.

I'm strong.

I show up.

I know that when things get rough, I don't cut and run.

These are facts I know about myself now.

I'm tenacious. And if something like cancer hurts me or my family? I strike back with everything I've got.

These are things I know about myself now that I didn't know before cancer. I suspected I could be strong. I thought I could be brave. Now, I know I am.

You will learn things about yourself, too. And I hope when people call you brave, you'll nod, bored, and say, "*I know.*"

You will know, in your bones, that you were tested and you came out the other side a champion. Those annoying people who dismissed you at the start with a "you've got this" and a shrug, were *right*, as irritating as that might be.

You will have earned that badge of honor, my friend. And one day, you will be the badass motherfucker in this club that no one ever wanted to join, welcoming in a new, petrified member. You'll be able to tell them it's all going to be okay. You'll be able to talk about your scars, your path and your journey.

Little Shit Is SO Little

The good news is that the stuff you obsessed about (your neighbor's ugly lawn gnomes, your coworker's smelly microwaved lunch) might actually not be so big anymore.

You faced fucking death.

You went through hell.

People getting worked up about who should be your home association's president feels. . . inconsequential.

You know why?

Because it is.

Cancer's silver lining is the gift of perspective. You know you have a limited time on this earth.

Every little hiccup in your life from now on, you'll compare it to cancer. Is it as bad as cancer? Probably not.

Hold on to that feeling. Don't let yourself get pulled back into petty bullshit. Remember that life is fleeting; do what you can to make whatever is left of yours count.

Lean into empathy.

Since you've walked through hell, you know how terrible life can get.

Use that life experience to be more empathetic to others. You might remember snapping the guy's head off at the drive-thru after getting bad biopsy results. You know all too well there are a lot of us out here having the worst day of their lives.

You know because you've been through it.

Your innate knowledge of this pain can help you be a beacon of light to others in a dark time.

The survivor's baton has been passed to you, and now YOU will be the veteran, the one others call on when they're first diagnosed. You'll be able to share your hard-fought wisdom. You'll be able to comfort others in your orbit.

I know this can feel scary. *You're* the expert now? Hell, yes, you are.

You're in the unique positions to help others the way other survivors have helped you.

And not just about cancer.

You can help family members or friends who are scared about something in their lives because you know how to let fear wash over you. You can be the guru in the lives of many because you're the veteran now. You've been to the battlefield and back. You have wisdom to share.

Now that you're healthy again, don't run scared from the experience. Some survivors I know want to bury this part of their lives and never look back at it. They want to run as fast as they can from the bleak moments and never relive them again. They can't wait to get back into the herd that never thinks about death.

I get that. I do.

They fear if they open that box, all that horrible, negative energy of that time will consume them.

But it won't.

But the past can't hurt you. It's not scary. You met the moment. You met it—scared, angry, however you were—but you met it. You dominated it. You survived.

That's not something to run from. It's something to be proud of. You DID it, my friend. You're alive. You may not have been a fucking gazelle, but you are a strong, motherfucking bull, who didn't back down.

You are glittering and goddess-like.

You are resilient.

You don't have to pity and pivot when your friends or family or spouse faces something hard. You can stare at the hard things in life with those you care about. You can hold their hands and see it together because you're not afraid.

What does this all mean, anyway?

While some want to stuff their cancer experience in a compartmentalized box and never open it again, others will try to make meaning out of it.

I read about one woman who was *sad* about being a survivor because she kept wondering what it was all for. She hadn't felt a calling like other women to form a charity, raise money for the cause, or do *anything* with her newfound lease on life. She worried she was wasting her second chance.

I'm here to tell you this: only you can find meaning in your struggle. And there may not be any meaning there. Or the meaning may come at a later time. You'll connect the dots or you won't, but you don't have to figure it all now. It's time to take the pressure off.

You don't have to make this a life-altering journey that shows you your true calling.

Or you can.

It's up to you.

Just like with how you handled cancer, there's no one right way.

Just like your cancer treatment was up to you—your decision—so are the lessons you learn and take away from your experience with cancer.

Do you become an advocate, shouting from the rooftops for people to get their mammograms? Or do you want to finally start that Etsy shop where you sell your pottery?

There's no right answer. There's just a right answer FOR YOU.

I was in the shower—where I do my best thinking and my very best crying—after my last immunotherapy treatment, when I decided to turn my cancer journal into this book. I came to a realization that a lot of the horrible moments in my life—including a miscarriage and then breast cancer—terribly traumatic events that were out of my control and seemed terribly unfair at the time, actually might have had a purpose after all.

I felt called during that shower to reach out and help others. You can assign whatever spiritual value you want to this, but it became clear to me that the moments in my life where I felt most abandoned by the universe were the times I was learning hard lessons about resilience that I could share with others.

You may or may not feel this calling, and that's okay.

It may not become clear to you—now or ever—why this happened to you. There may not be a reason. We can't explain everything.

Or maybe you just need this extra time so you can love others. So you can comfort friends. So you can be your best self.

Give yourself grace in this time. Go back and enjoy the things in your life you couldn't before (for me this was cheese and coffee!). You don't have to have an epiphany now or ever. You don't have to talk about this time ever again. Or you can talk about it all the time. This experience can bring you more in touch with your faith and spirituality or less.

The choice—as it always has been—is yours.

We're all living on bonus time.

The thing about fighting off a deadly disease is that if you're so lucky as to end treatment and go into remission, every single healthy minute after that is bonus time.

The road back to normal (if there ever was such a thing) is long and twisty. We'll have difficult days post-treatment, frustrating days, when we're disillusioned and fed up, as we all get sometimes, when we're paying bills, trying to slash debt, bumping heads with a new boss, or getting crossways with our spouse, our best friend, or our kids. We'll start to think: *why does everything have to be so hard? I've already DONE hard, and I'm so, so very tired of hard...*

When this happens, I tell myself... this is bonus time.

I wasn't, even, technically supposed to be here at all.

The cancer growing in me was a countdown clock. If I'd never gotten that mammogram, or if I'd turned down treatment, well, the clock would've run out on me. That would be it. Life over. Early, as it happens, at 51 or 52.

I wouldn't be here.

So right now, every minute, every hour of healthy life, well, it's bonus time.

Bonus time won't always be easy. It won't always be fun. But the true gift is having the time at all.

Keep up those healthy habits.

You may never make sense of why cancer happened to you, or how to make it meaningful in your life, but you can take the hardest won lessons from this fight into your future.

- **Lower your tolerance for bullshit.** Worry less about the little stuff—because unless you're facing fucking cancer and death, it's all little shit.
- **Self-care is essential.** You've had good practice taking care of yourself through chemo, post-surgery, and the like. Keep doing it. Have your own back. You know you can do it now. Keep doing it. The more you take care of yourself, the better and kinder you'll be to others.
- **Be kind to yourself.** Stop that negative playlist in your head.
- **Empathize more than ever.** You've suffered, and you can see others suffering. You know how hard it is, and you also know how much a kind word meant to you—even from a stranger at the grocery store—when you needed it most. Pay it forward now.

You've faced death. Your mettle has been challenged in this fundamental way, and you've risen to the occasion. Other people haven't faced this. They might be obsessed with the Little Shit, and you can't even understand why.

You, my friend, have climbed Mount Everest in flip-flops and made it to the summit. You didn't think you'd make it, did you? But you did.

I knew you would. I always knew you would.

You didn't believe me when I told you that at the beginning of this book, did you? But I knew you had it in you. I knew you'd do well in this badass club. I know you'd fit right in.

I'm sorry you had to join us.

I hope one day we cure cancer and this club is closed to new members forever. I'd like nothing more than for no one to ever have to read this book again except in history class when people have to study this weird, deadly disease called "cancer" that's now a relic of the past.

Until then, let me say, I'm glad you're here. I'm proud of you and how far you've come.

Now, you can now live in the moment, make whatever bonus time is left in your life matter to you.

One Final Pep Talk:

Hello, Golden Warrior.

You really don't need any more pep talks.

You are a goddess who has kicked cancer's ass (or will soon). Go forth in your life with the confidence of a woman who has faced her greatest fears and conquered them. You are a full-fledged member of the Club of Bad Asses. You have earned your bravery medal. When people say, "You're so brave," in your heart you'll know they're right. You ARE brave.

Because cancer tried to scare you into inaction, terrify you into sitting down and giving up. But you didn't. You deserve the Didn't Quit medal because you keep on going—one step, one cry, one stumble at a time. You kept on going. Not everyone did. Not everyone will. But YOU did.

You showed up.

For your family. Your friends. For yourself.

You walked through the fire, my friend. You climbed that mountain in fucking flip-flops. You stared death in the face, and you laughed.

You know you're tough. You KNOW you're resilient.

I know how hard this battle has been.

Your scars are your badges of honor. Wear them with pride.

In this battle, you are a survivor. You are no victim.

CARA LOCKWOOD

I want you to know that this battle is part of you, but it does not define you.

You define you.

What you do next is up to you.

Acknowledgments

I'm alive today thanks to the hard work, love, and prayers of an army of amazing soldiers who fought this battle shoulder-to-shoulder with me.

First and foremost, I must thank my amazing husband, PJ, who stood by me and fought giants, never letting me go into that scary white room alone. I want to thank my kids: Hana, Miya, Pete, Sarina, and Sophia, who battled right along with me and shared the stress. Cancer effects everyone. Thank you to Sarina for helping me with the book cover's graphic design. To my husband and kids—thank you for giving me the very best reasons to live: you.

To other members of my family: Mom, Dad, Patty, Matt, Jill, Rodney, Artie, Olga, and so many more for having my back, and for making me feel loved and cared for.

I have so many friends to thank—Shannon, my ride or die, who sent me gifts every single week of treatment. To Hillary, Gretchen, Dani, Julie, Annie, Johnny, Atorina, Beth Kinsella AND Beth Zadick, who kept the meal train going, and to Stina, Stacey, Carroll, Linda, and Patti for all the support. To all the neighbors on my street (Shirley, Gary, Rosemary, Bill, and everyone else) who checked in on me or dropped off goodies, thank you. To the prayer chains (there were many), thank you. To Jordana who picked up volunteer alumni fundraising slack – thank you. To them and all of my other amazing friends who never pitied and pivoted, a huge, heartfelt thank you.

I want to thank my medical team at Northwestern Medicine. Dr. Mary Ahn, my breast surgeon, Dr. Lauren Fischer, my plastic surgeon, Dr. Ami Shah, my oncologist. I want to thank Erica, the RN in Dr. Fischer's office who helped me understand reconstruction, eased my fears, and was always and forever a trustworthy source of the best information. Thank you, Danielle, in Dr. Ahn's office, for helping me find sooner MRIs and other diagnostic testing sites.

I want to thank ALL my amazing nurse navigators who kept the schedules running, and everyone at the Warrenville Cancer Center, as well as the army of physician assistants, nurses, medical aids, nutritionists, physical therapists, geneticists, cancer researchers, and volunteers. Special shout-out to my very first amazing chemotherapy nurse there who went out of her way to even come to a book signing. Not only did she ease my fears on that first day, she also helped me believe I really could do the treatment when I wasn't at all sure I could. You are an angel among angels. Thank you.

I want to thank the staff at Central DuPage Hospital, where I got my double mastectomy, and Delnor Community Hospital, where I got diagnostic testing. I'd like to thank the Breast Clinic in Glen Ellyn, where I got my mammogram and diagnosis.

I want to thank the Living Well Cancer Center for giving me a free wig, massages, support groups and more.

I want to thank Mark Gurda, who helped me get insurance, and the Affordable Care Act, which outlawed pre-existing conditions (because, otherwise, I would've never gotten insurance when my COBRA ran out).

I'd like to thank my talented counselor, Victoria Baum, who helped me get my head right for the fight.

I'd like to thank the breast cancer beta readers, Karen Preston, Claire, Jenny, and everyone else!

Thank you to Wasabi Publicity for helping me get the word out about this book.

I'd also like to thank all the fellow members of the breast cancer warrior club—I'm in awe of YOU all, every day, and it's an honor to be in this group with you. Thank you to every single badass member of this club for showing me the way.

Thank you to all the amazing charities out there—Susan G. Komen, the Breast Cancer Research Foundation, and many more—working hard to support warriors and to cure cancer. Let's all work together to make sure no one actually ever needs to read this book ever again.

www.ingramcontent.com/pod-product-compliance
Lightning Source LLC
Chambersburg PA
CBHW031459270326
41930CB00006B/168